No, they won't 'just sound like each other'

DUISBURGER ARBEITEN ZUR SPRACH- UND KULTURWISSENSCHAFT

Duisburg Papers on Research in Language and Culture

Herausgegeben von
Ulrich Ammon, René Dirven und Martin Pütz

Band 72

PETER LANG
Frankfurt am Main · Berlin · Bern · Bruxelles · New York · Oxford · Wien

Laura Sicola

No, they won't 'just sound like each other'

NNS-NNS Negotiated Interaction and Attention to Phonological Form on Targeted L2 Pronunciation Tasks

PETER LANG
Internationaler Verlag der Wissenschaften

Bibliographic Information published by the Deutsche Nationalbibliothek

The Deutsche Nationalbibliothek lists this publication in the Deutsche Nationalbibliografie; detailed bibliographic data is available in the internet at <http://www.d-nb.de>.

ISSN 0934-3709
ISBN 978-3-631-58476-7

www.peterlang.de

Dedicated to all language teachers and learners
who are out there doing the things academics write about.

ACKNOWLEDGEMENTS

There are many people without whose help this dissertation would never have been realized. To begin with, I would like to thank the members of my dissertation committee. First, Dr. Teresa Pica, the chair of my committee, has been a mentor for the past seven years. Her academic and professional guidance has been invaluable, and her untiring willingness and ability to answer e-mail inquiries at any hour of the day or night is a testament to her dedication to the field. Dr. Mary Ann Julian has also been a constant source of support, first by hiring me to teach ESL at the university, then overseeing my data collection as a committee member, collaborating on graduate course instruction as a colleague, and helping me see it all through to the end. Finally, to Dr. William Poser, who took a unique interest in the applied nature of my work, and supervised the accuracy of the phonological arguments herein (though any remaining inaccuracies are solely my own.)

In addition to my committee, I would like to thank the teachers at the English Language Programs who allowed me to use their class time to conduct the study and the students who agreed to participate; the graduate students who helped with the early stages of raw transcription; and in particular my fellow PhD candidates, Jiyoon Lee and Shannon Sauro, who dedicated so much time to on round after round of coding revisions.

Special thanks go to Dr. Martin Pütz, who believed in my work enough to take a chance on me, and gave me the unique opportunity to publish this dissertation through Peter Lang Publishers.

Finally, I must thank my family and friends who have stood by me and encouraged me through all of the ups and downs of this journey, resisting the urge to ask, "Aren't you done yet?" Now I can finally tell them: Yes, I am. But in truth, the journey is just beginning.

Laura Sicola
September, 2008

TABLE OF CONTENTS

LIST OF TABLES

LIST OF FIGURES

CHAPTER 1

STATEMENT OF THE PROBLEM

INTRODUCTION

This study has evolved out of more than a decade of personal experience and interest in teaching second or foreign language for communicative competence. Of all aspects of second and foreign language development, pronunciation[1] is arguably the most elusive, and potentially the most contentious theoretically and pedagogically. Over the years, questions pertaining to foreign accents and pronunciation have been widely debated. What is an "accent?" What makes it regional or foreign, intelligible or unintelligible? Can pronunciation be taught and/or learned, and for that matter, should it? The prevailing perspective at any given time has had significant influence on the extent and manner in which pronunciation is incorporated into L2 pedagogical approaches (1997; Morley, 1991, 1994; Pennington & Richards, 1986). Yet student preferences have consistently indicated that they give pronunciation a high priority (Macdonald, Yule, & Powers, 1994). Indeed, research over the last two decades or so has shown what many have believed all along: that "*intelligible pronunciation is an essential component of communicative competence*" (Morley, 1991).

The ubiquitous question, then, remains how best to help learners improve their intelligibility. Pennington and Richards (1986) summarize the complexity of the challenge: "[t]he development of L2 phonology can be viewed as a dynamic *process* involving cognitive, psychomotor, linguistic, and interactive factors" (p.214) and as a result, "[a]rticulatory, interactional, and cognitive *processes* are all equally involved" (p.212, emphasis mine). Yet on many levels these *processes* are still awaiting exploration in research and practice alike. Thus, the purpose of this dissertation is to take a first step towards discovering how learners cognitively process L2 phonological data, in order to shed light on how help them reach their goal of attaining communicative competence.

Historically, many pedagogical approaches and curricula have been created in attempt to help language learners reach more targetlike pronunciation and phonological perception abilities, yet little success has been documented in research or practice. In fact, most teachers can give numerous examples of students who have demonstrated noticeable improvement in their overall fluency and accuracy in most areas of language, but little to no change in their

---

1 Although *pronunciation* can generally be viewed as a set of skills, and *phonology* is traditionally viewed as an abstract system of sounds, in this paper, *pronunciation* and *phonology* will be used interchangeably unless otherwise specified, with both referring to sound patterns of a language to be productively and receptively acquired.

pronunciation (Snow & Hoefnagel-Höhle, 1979, as cited in Markham, 1997, p. 22).[2] However, in the past three decades, ever-growing bodies of research in second language acquisition (SLA) have investigated the potential roles of cognitive processes such as attention and noticing in facilitating L2 development. In part, this may have been in response to Hatch's early call for researchers to examine interaction "as a basis for examining the linguistic and cognitive features of the L2 Learning process" (Pica, 1994). Today, this function remains as potentially valuable—yet not nearly as widely explored—for understanding L2 phonological acquisition as for other areas of L2 learning. To date, L2 processing research has commonly sought to identify what forms learners naturally attend to, or more narrowly how and when learners may attend to certain lexical or morphosyntactic forms, but the acquisitional processing of phonological forms has been all but excluded from extensive, specific discussion in the field of SLA. This occurs in spite of the fact that cognition-oriented studies in SLA have found that learners will naturally attend to pronunciation problems that cause a breakdown in communication, just as they will attend to problems of lexis or (in some cases more than) morphosyntax.

Repercussions of this oversight are three-fold: First, the generalizability of hypotheses regarding L2 processing and language learning is necessarily limited due to their lack of testing in the prominent sub-field of interlanguage phonology (ILPh). Second, little more is known now than 25 years ago about how learners process L2 phonological data. Third, there has been little intent or opportunity for L2 pronunciation research and practice to inform each other, since there has been little to no research on the role of processing in pronunciation learning. As a result, current pedagogy has been left to rely heavily on antiquated methodologies and much intuition, some of which is mutually contradicting. L2 research and pedagogy are beginning to have greater influence on each other with regard to areas such as morphosyntactic and lexical development (see Doughty & Williams, 1998, all), and so it is timely that similar changes should be made with regard to pronunciation. As a result, it is necessary for SLA research to begin answering the many calls to explore how learners process L2 phonological data (Ellis, 1999a; Hansen, 2004; Marinis, 2003; Morley, 1991; Pennington, 1998; Pennington & Richards, 1986; Williams, 2005). Thus, the primary goal of this dissertation will be to explore cognitive processing in L2 phonological development by extending the methods and findings of research on other areas of L2 developmental processing into this

2 "The Joseph Conrad phenomenon" is a label sometimes given to the extreme of this condition, referring to the famous British author of Polish descent, Joseph Conrad, who started learning English as a teenager, and wrote with perfectly nativelike English vocabulary, grammar, and stylistic discourse, yet retained a heavy Polish accent despite decades of living in Britain as an adult. Henry Kissinger, German-born US secretary of State from 1973-1977 is another frequently referenced example (Han, 2004)

area, and the secondary goal will be to identify potential applicability of the results to L2 pronunciation pedagogy.

This chapter will provide the theoretical framework for the study. First, it will give an overview of the predominantly representational, product-oriented research that has been undertaken to explore L2 pronunciation. The evidence will show that the next logical step is to look at how learners cognitively process L2 phonological data. The subsequent section will outline what has been identified as a potential role of attention in SLA as a component of cognitive processing of language code and meaning. Finally, this chapter will review some of the possible ways in which researching how learners attend to L2 phonological forms as a possible preliminary step in the acquisition of L2 pronunciation would pose a challenge to the field. This will lead to a call to take a new process orientation to the definition and measurement of *learning* in L2 pronunciation, rather than continuing to define and measure *learning* in strict terms of a language product.

State and Status in L2 Pronunciation Research

Can adult learners successfully learn to perceive and produce the sound system of a second or foreign language? Typically, research regarding L2 pronunciation has attempted to examine, describe, and explain phonological patterns in learners' interlanguage based on the interaction of three key factors: the L1, the L2, and language universals (Major, 2001). SLA research and theoretical linguistics have addressed the potential balance between access to universal grammar (UG) and the influence of the L1 in helping and hindering many aspects of L2 development, including phonology. Although some early researchers argued that adult learners would always retain negative L1 phonological influences in the L2 (Scovel, 1969), since then others have argued that L1 transfer can have a positive role in SLA (Corder, 1993) and that adult learners do have at least some access to principles of UG (see Ioup & Weinberger, 1987; Major, 2001; Markham, 1997, for comprehensive reviews). The issues of L1 transfer and potential for UG access will be discussed below.

The approaches have followed the trends in phonological theory (Eckman, 2004; Major, 2001), in which focus has typically been to identify and describe theoretical rules or constraints of the "accent" (i.e. the phonetic product) and explain the manifestation of these patterns. More recently, these linguistic theories have begun to converge with SLA theory and attempted to explain what other factors may have caused them, may have caused them to change over time, have caused them to vary from learner to learner or to vary within a single learner's speech. Archibald notes that reasons for accent "may be phonologically-, phonetically-, perceptually-, or motorically-based" (1998, pp. 23-33). Han (2004) provides an extensive compilation of studies exploring factors that influence L2 fossilization on the whole, most of which pertain directly to or at least hold implications for phonological development, or cessation thereof. This section will identify some of the common and most relevant themes in the factors explored in research on L2 phonology (for more comprehensive reviews, see Eckman, 1994; Markham, 1997; Major, 2001), including transfer, learner characteristics, instruction, and task-specific conditions, specifically formality and the influence of orthography. The evidence indicating potential for interlanguage phonological restructuring will be presented, which will lead to an essential, emergent question: How and when do such changes occur?

L1 Transfer as a factor

There are several prominent areas of research that have attempted to identify influential linguistic factors of L2 pronunciation. The role of L1 transfer has been discussed for decades (Gass & Selinker, 1993). Studies have consistently shown that the learner's L1 is a powerful influence on the specific features of a learner's interlanguage pronunciation, even more so than on interlanguage syntax (Ellis, 1994) although not all speakers of a shared L1 will demonstrate transfer of the same phonological forms into a shared L2. The Contrastive Analysis Hypothesis (CAH) (Lado, 1957) proposed that areas (phonological or otherwise) in which the L1 and L2 differ will cause difficulty for learners, and the Markedness Differential Hypothesis (MDH) (Eckman 1977, 1987) takes the predictability a step further by asserting that "difficulty" is relative to universals of markedness, in that components of the L2 will be more difficult – but not necessarily impossible – to acquire if they are not only different but also more marked than the L1, whereas L2 forms that are different but less marked than the L1 form will not be difficult to learn. Flege and MacKay support Flege's Speech Learning Model (SLM) (e.g. Flege 1988, 1995) which asserts that adults do indeed retain (at least some) access to UG capacities that enable perception of L2 sounds and establishment of new L2 phonetic categories (2004). The SLM looks not so much at markedness, but at perceived similarity, and explains that the less similar an L2 sound is perceived to be to the closest L1 sound, the more likely it is to be noticed by the learner, and subsequently assigned its own phonetic category. Minimally, at least some phonetic difference must be noticed for a new category to be established. This conclusion leads one to ask why some contrasts are noticed more easily than others, and if it is possible to assist learners in noticing them. An approach to investigating the role of *noticing* will be addressed in greater depth later in this chapter. Ultimately, phonological theory research suggests that despite the influence of L1, adult learners do have the ability to reset their IL parameters to conform to L2 settings (see Archibald, 1998, for a thorough discussion and critique), and that noticing may play an important role in this resetting.

Instruction as a factor

Studies pertaining to effects of both quantity and quality of instruction on L2 pronunciation are comparatively scarce, and far from consistent in target, population, research design or instructional approach (Pennington & Richards, 1986), but preliminary indications are that learners may be able to attain more targetlike perception and production with the help of narrowly focused instructional intervention. In her review of L2 pronunciation studies, Pennington (1998) recognized that most successful learners had studied pronunciation separately from other areas of language development. There is also evidence to show that learners who have attained strongly targetlike pronunciation often have also received explicit articulatory or perceptually-based training and correction, stressing L1-L2 contrasts when possible (Bongaerts, 1999; de Bot, 1980; de Bot & Malifert, 1982; Pennington, 1998).

Studies of comparative instructional approaches such as traditional drill-and-practice, self-study with cassettes, or no instruction (Macdonald et al., 1994) or form-focused instruction vs. meaning-focused or forms-and-meaning-focused instruction (Park, 2000) have typically not identified any significant short- or long-term effects for any particular type of instruction. However, the lack of effect may have been due to design issues rather than the value of the instructional approach itself. These and other comparative instruction studies have tended to be holistic in their evaluation of learners' pronunciation, rather than controlling for the number of phonemes or prosodic features to be addressed, which may have influenced their findings. Perhaps tighter limitations on learning objectives would have yielded more telling results.

What most of the intervention studies share are data collections taken pre- and post-intervention, in attempt to measure and compare accuracy of some aspects of learners' speech performance. What may prove more enlightening at this point is to look at what happens *during* the comparative interventions to check for evidence of learning at the moment that it happens. This would be a logical and potentially valuable next step in assessing the effects of instructional intervention on L2 pronunciation development, and is a strong motivation of the current study.

Learner characteristics as factors

Piske, MacKay and Flege (2001) summarize much of the literature on ILPh and identify the most commonly explored factors, such as age of learning (AO), length of residence in the L2 environment (LOR), the amount and/or type of formal L2 instruction received, and other common categories such as "motivation, language learning aptitude and amount of L1/L2 use" (p. 195). For the purposes of this study, in this section, maturational constraints (i.e. age), and motivation will be briefly reviewed, as they have most frequently been attributed with having direct effects on a learner's ability and willingness to restructure his or her ILPh, respectively.

Maturational constraints

Are adults biologically capable of learning the sound system of a new language? Age, and its relative maturational constraints, is generally viewed as one of the most critical determinants of ultimate attainment in L2 pronunciation. Han (2004) identified this factor as one of the two strongest influences in SLA, along with L1 transfer, that can "predispose adult L2 learners to fossilization" (p. 167). The argued point partially hinges on whether lateralization of cerebral hemispheres – generally completed by puberty – results in a loss of neuroplasticity and accessibility to compartmentalized functions, limiting further potential for linguistic development. It is generally presumed that all but the most exceptional learners will retain a non-native accent if they begin learning the target language after childhood (Oyama, 1976).

While the original Critical Period Hypothesis (CPH) (Lenneberg, 1967) was intended to indicate age constraints on L1 learning, the potential existence of several sensitive periods for various domains of L2 development has been widely discussed,[3] with pronunciation abilities generally believed to be the most susceptible to an early sensitive period.[4] (See Han, 2004; Markham, 1997; Major, 2001, for overviews of the biological arguments supporting and refuting the existence of critical and sensitive periods.) However, adults have demonstrated ability to do as well or better than children or adolescents in the short term and on certain tasks (Snow & Hoefnagel-Höhle, 1978). Biological studies have yet to provide conclusive evidence regarding ultimate phonological limitations pertaining to age, and claims grow more questionable with each individual adult learner who seems to have defied the odds and passed for native (Markham, 1997; Neufeld, 2001).

The exact age that delimits this critical or sensitive period remains in question, whether as early as age five or six, or as late as the end of puberty (for reviews of claims, see Archibald, 1998; Han, 2004; Major, 2001; Markham, 1997). Nevertheless, there is ample evidence to show that adult learners, despite

---

3 Han (2004) justifies use of the terms "critical period" and "sensitive period" interchangeably with regard to SLA. For the purposes of this paper, however, the term "critical period" will be used to imply absolute limitations, and "sensitive period" will be used to indicate a more flexible, non-absolute period pertaining to L2 learning potential, as per Oyama (1976), unless referring to L1 or otherwise specified.

4 This emphasis on pronunciation limitations over grammatical or lexical limitations is partially due to the fact that "'sound patterns are produced by actual motor activity and are thus directly initiated by neurophysiological mechanisms' and 'lexical and syntactic patterns lack any such "neurophysiological reality"' (Scovel, 1969: 252)" (Han, 2004) The physical and physiological nature of pronunciation and phonological development will be discussed in chapter 2.

having long past any chronological sensitive period, do have the ability to develop more targetlike L2 pronunciation; as Markham summarizes, "neither age nor experience appear to reliably predict the perception, classification, and production of sounds (1997, p. 129). Of equal consequence is the finding that although fossilization may be inevitable at some point, "it can be modulated (aggravated or alleviated) by environmental, social and psychological forces" (Han, 2004, p. 43.) Most importantly, with implications for pedagogy and this study, "(s)everal studies have shown that *cognitive strategies* can influence lateralization" (Archibald, 1998, p. 21; emphasis in original). The issue of cognition and SLA will be discussed later in this chapter. Thus, it is likely that age-related influences on L2 pronunciation are at best indicative of a flexible sensitive period, not an absolute critical period, and can be influenced by external stimuli.

Motivation as a factor

The term *motivation* will be used broadly here, encompassing any social-psychological factor that influences the degree to which a learner strives to master or resist use of the L2's phonological system. Studies of motivation in L2 in general have been well documented for decades (Crookes & Schmidt, 1991; Gardner & Lambert, 1972; Schumann, 1976; Zuengler, 1989), generally finding positive correlation between motivation and L2 success, though studies specifically geared towards the correlation between L2 pronunciation and motivation are less conclusive (Markham, 1997). At the most basic level, the only guarantee, per se, is that any learner who deliberately chooses to *resist* learning or employing L2 phonological rules, such as those wishing to be clearly identified as a member of their L1 communities at all times, will *not* progress towards native-like L2 pronunciation. On the other hand, learners are more likely to attempt to accommodate the target language behaviors including pronunciation in order to communicate successfully and/or "fit in" with a particular group of speakers of the L2. However, they are less likely to make additional effort to change their speech patterns if they feel that their current communicative needs are being met, and their messages are being successfully received by their interlocutor (Han, 2004), and that they are socially accepted.

Markham's (1997) Achievement Model of Phonetic Acquisition (AMPA) posits that the learner's "imitative base" and "imitative skill complex" are the fundamental determinants of a learner's phonological potential, but that the ego-permeability, or sense of identity, and other affective qualities as the two other major factors that "impose themselves on the degree to which he can exploit his skills to greatest effect" (p. 131). Although it is not clear if strong motivation will predispose a learner to attain more accurate L2 perception or production abilities, the general understanding is that a shared quality among successful L2 learners with more targetlike pronunciation is a strong motivation to improve these particular skills (Bongaerts, 1999; Pennington, 1998). The positive implications held for learners, instructors and researchers alike is that since ego, affect, and other motivational factors are at least partially responses to *external conditions*, the likelihood of any positive effects thereof can potentially be increased by manipulating the conditions themselves (Markham, 1997).

Task conditions as factors

There are myriad task[5] conditions that can and do influence the accuracy of learners' pronunciation. While a comprehensive discussion thereof is beyond the scope of this investigation, two will be discussed here, task formality and orthography, based on their prominence in and unique application to L2 phonological research, respectively. What is important to note is that these factors can influence the perception and production tendencies of a single learner from moment to moment. This *intralearner* variability will ultimately be presented as a starting point and justification for studying adult learners' potential to acquire L2 sounds as a step toward ultimately attaining greater intelligibility and communicative competence.

Task formality[6]

It is generally uncontested that the formality of a task will influence the carefulness of the speech, and thereby influence the accuracy of a learner's L2 pronunciation, specifically that the accuracy will be in direct relationship to the formality (Archibald, 1998; Major, 1987; Tarone, 1983, 1987). Simply put, "(t)he more formal the style, the more a speaker can eliminate interference processes because he or she is paying more attention to form" (Major, 1987). This is held to be as true for pronunciation as for other areas of L2 production. The potential role of attention to form in SLA theory will be discussed later in this chapter.

Task formality can influence the linguistic and compensatory strategies used by students. For example, task formality is linked to linguistically compensatory strategies such as epenthesis and deletion. This is seen in studies of recoverability (Weinberger, 1987) which demonstrate evidence of the influence of task formality on intralearner variation in the ratio of epenthesis or deletion of L2 codas. Weinberger (1987) points out the role of context, and explains that interlanguage phonological forms may surface in ways that create an ambiguity

5 In phonological research, both L1 and L2, the word "task" is not operationalized the same way it is in SLA research, most notably in Pica, Kanagy and Falodun's (1993) classifications of "communicative task types." This latter work will be discussed in greater detail in chapter 2.

6 In phonological research, a "formal" task is generally one that is tightly controlled with little linguistic context, such as the reading aloud of word lists or minimal pairs, and does not necessarily correspond to sociolinguistic formality of speech style or register, etc.

of meaning, such as by deletion of codas, and that ultimately the underlying form must be recoverable through the linguistic environment. Epenthesis, in contrast, preserves the underlying form and avoids ambiguity more easily than deletion if there isn't any context from which to derive the meaning, as is the case with formal elicitation tasks. This is evident in such cases as (a) below:

(a) "cat" /kæt/ -->[kætə] vs. [kæ]
"cap" /kæp/-->[kæpə] vs. [kæ]

He demonstrated a correlation between the degree of task formality and compensatory strategy: specifically, learners were more likely to use epenthesis in formal tasks such as reading word lists or minimal pair tasks, with no linguistic contexts, where a pair such as "cat" and "cap" as seen above, would otherwise be rendered indistinguishable by deletion, and successful communication of meaning would be lost. In contrast, interviews or other less formal tasks allowed learners to delete codas and place the onus on the listener to recover the underlying word form and communicative meaning from contextual information. In essence, these strategic choices are examples of what a task is capable of eliciting from a learner. If this is true, then it implies that learners can become aware of when they need to modify their pronunciation to preserve meaning. Whether the awareness can be externally triggered, the point at which the awareness occurs, and how learners subsequently decide what modification to make to their pronunciation are questions that need to be explored.

Orthography

Another task-related influence in learners' varied accuracy in segmental production, which has been more closely explored in the past 15 years or so, is the presence or absence of orthographic cues. On the more positive side, learners may associate mortoric pattern differences in the physical articulation of the [l] and [r], for example, and thus produce more targetlike distinctions between 'lake' and 'rake' when reading aloud than when using either or both words freely in extemporaneous speech when no such visual orthographic cues are available. One problem with this strategy is that learner's orthography-articulation connection may bypass the learner's true underlying phonological representation (Flege, et al., 1995 and Brown, 1997, as cited in Archibald, 1998). In other words, the learner may not truly recognize the phonological difference between the two sounds, which also may be evident if a learner's ability to perceive a phonetic contrast is less accurate than his or her production thereof.

On the other hand, orthographic cues can also potentially have the opposite effect, causing more transfer-based errors if a learner associates a letter or symbol with a specific sound from the L1,[7] especially in such cases as cognates (Markham, 1997), and the inclination to assign a sound to every letter. Such tendencies can cause less targetlike production than would be observed in a task that relied less heavily on written cues (Archibald, 1998). (For a more thorough explanation of the effects of orthography on pronunciation, see Markham, 1997). Thus, researchers and practitioners must bear orthographic influence in mind when designing elicitation materials and tasks, and find ways to make learners aware of both the potential problems and resources therein.

Phonology section conclusion

This section has attempted to show that research in L2 phonological theory provides evidence that adult language learners do retain some underlying capacity to acquire L2 phonological forms. The existence of intralearner variation in pronunciation seems to be one of the greatest indicators that adults should be able to modify their speech, at least within their own range of less-targetlike to more-targetlike sounds. Since their most targetlike production is an indicator of what they are linguistically and physically capable of producing, at least under certain conditions, it can be hypothesized that a learner's least targetlike pronunciation should be able to improve at least to the quality of his or her most targetlike uses.

Only since the early 1990s have linguists begun to consider how learning is triggered, and attempt to incorporate learning theory into UG models of acquisition. However, most phonological theories share "an explicit concern with *representation* as opposed to *process*," i.e. identifying the structures – and factors that may account for the identified structures – rather than *how* the structures change (Archibald, 1998). The next step is to delve deeper into how and when phonological components are actually learned to some degree, which may be possible by borrowing methods from SLA to explore cognitive processes involved in language development. Attention and noticing, two of the most prominently researched processes in SLA, will be discussed in the next section.

Cognitive Processing and Attention to Form in SLA Research

The Role of Attention

The role of attention in SLA has been debated for the last 25 years, although most theories acknowledge that attention, particularly conscious attention in the sense of awareness, to a particular linguistic form will likely facilitate a learner's

7 I have noticed this phenomenon in my own studies of Japanese as a foreign language over the years. When reading Japanese text aloud, I am uncomfortably aware of a noticeably stronger American accent if the text is written in the Romanized script (*romaji*) than if it is written in one of the traditional Japanese syllabaries (*katakana* or *hiragana*) or the Chinese-based ideographs, *kanji*. I am also aware that it is harder for me to "turn off" my accent as I read *romaji*, despite conscious efforts in the moment.

processing of that form as a step towards its acquisition. Schmidt asserts that "SLA is largely driven by what learners pay attention to and notice in the target language input and what they understand the significance of noticed input to be" (2001, pp. 3-4). Thus, it is essential that learners be able to pay attention to and notice target language pronunciation elements, and that they understand the communicative value these elements carry.

Attention has many related psychological processes and functions, including awareness, noticing, and detection, all of which overlap in ways that have yet to be fully delimited. This section will identify relevant interpretations of the relationships between the key components necessary to understand the role of attention to form in SLA as it would potentially facilitate development of ILPh.

Attention to form can be viewed as the driving force behind SLA because it is the mediating factor that determines what L2 input data is made available for further processing, and what passes by without registering, whether lexical, morphosyntactic, pragmatic, or phonological. However, as *attention* has been inconsistently operationalized as related to *noticing* and *awareness*, for the purposes of this study Tomlin and Villa's (1994) model will be used as a basis due to its applicability to research and pedagogy alike. According to their model, when a form catches the learner's attention, it may undergo at least three levels of the attending process. The first is ***alertness***, or a simple readiness to receive input, which could simply mean that the person is not daydreaming or is prepared to listen. More importantly, their second level of attention is ***orientation,*** which is an alignment (voluntary or involuntary) of attentional resources towards specific input data, i.e. "heightened sensitivity to a specific feature of some incoming stimulus" (p. 197). Thus, orienting the learner's attention to a form can serve to precondition their receptivity towards it, and thus facilitate other acquisitional processes. Learners can be independently oriented toward a particular form, or an external force can trigger the orientation, such as a teacher prefacing a lesson with a suggestion to listen for a particular form. Orientation is viewed as being facilitative, though not always essential. However, it is the third level, ***detection***, on which acquisition ultimately occurs, because it is here that "cognitive registration of sensory stimuli" happens, which is a necessary prerequisite for additional subsequent processing (p.192-193). The complicated nature of detection requires further clarification as it relates to noticing and awareness.

Robinson (2001a) distinguishes between two types of detection: with and without the construct of awareness, where *awareness* is defined as "conscious perception or noticing" (p. 18). As he also defines *noticing* as "detection plus rehearsal in short-term memory, prior to encoding in long-term memory" (p. 296), then noticing necessarily implies an element of consciousness in registration of input data in working memory as a potentially necessary precursor to long-term memory storage, whether the rehearsal is internally processed or outwardly manifested verbally. Schmidt (1995) explains that without noticing, i.e. without conscious awareness, detection could simply be called "registration," (p.18) and is useful, but only for facilitating processing of structures that previously were established. In contrast, it is the very act of noticing that is the "necessary and sufficient condition for the conversion of input to intake for learning" (Schmidt, 1994, p. 17, as cited in Bitchener, 2004), where *intake* is the "portion of the available input that is selectively attended to and extracted from the stream of speech for further processing" (Doughty, 2001, p. 214), or more succinctly, "the detection, processing, and storage of input" (Philp, 2003, p. 101). It is through this process of attention to form that noticing can facilitate intake as one of the preliminary cognitive processes necessary for SLA.

However, while most targeted studies on attention, noticing and intake have been carried out on morphosyntactic or lexical forms, the study of phonological forms has not been undertaken in this way. Thus, L2 phonological acquisition "needs to be reconceptualized at the [...] cognitive [and other] levels" (Pennington, 1998, p. 337.) To this end, this study extends a cognitive approach to the study of interlanguage phonological development in light of the contributions that this attention-oriented approach has made to the understanding of L2 structural and lexical development.

Challenges of Researching the Acquisition of L2 Pronunciation

A key challenge to instruction and research of L2 pronunciation learning is that, more so than vocabulary and grammar, interlearner variability ranges in the extremes as far as the accuracy of one's production and perception of L2 sounds from the moment of the first utterance, regardless of age, L1, or other factors commonly accepted as being influential in L2 pronunciation. As Major explains, "in morphology and syntax if the L2 speaker knows the NS target, then it will be achieved," whereas "[i]n L2 phonology the possibilities are more complicated [...] because the output is not so directly linked to the intention as it is in syntax and morphology" (Major, 2001). Thus, L2 pronunciation learning requires learners to identify similarities and differences in the IL and target language (TL) inventories in order to add non-overlapping L2 sounds to the learner's IL and replace L1 and IL sound patterns that have been systematic substitutes. As a result of the near-immediate establishment of an ILPh and the need to modify it to become more targetlike, learners must be able to "notice the gap" (Schmidt & Frota, 1986; Swain, 1985, 1998) between target language phonological input and their own ILPh. The inherent value in this particular type of noticing is that it can "destabilize the IL and move it toward more targetlike accuracy, a later stage in acquisition" (Williams, 2005, p. 682). Making these changes represents the basis of what Markham refers to as phonological and phonetic acquisition (1997). He distinguishes *phonological acquisition* as development of a system of abstract categories of perception and production, and the degrees of permissible variation thereof, and *phonetic acquisition* as demonstration of these categories in surface performance (1997, p. 16).

This "gap" can be particularly challenging for NNSs to notice independently, since some phonological forms in certain contexts can lack perceptual salience for learners. Alternatively, NNSs may recognize a difference, but not perceive it as being necessary to successfully communicate meaning. In my own experience, when I speak in Spanish with friends from Barcelona, I can clearly hear a difference, or "gap," between the way they pronounce /s/ in most words[8] and the way I pronounce /s/, though I cannot yet produce it as they do, and presume based on uninterrupted conversation that my articulation is "close enough" to allow meaning to be successfully conveyed. Other learners may possess the metalinguistic knowledge regarding the existence of the /θ/ or the /l/-/r/ contrast, for example, and may even be physically capable of perceiving and producing the sounds on command, but do not perceive any communicative necessity for the regular inclusion thereof.

Thus, interlocutors may play an essential role in helping NNSs identify the gap by indicating a lack of comprehension, whereby drawing the learner's attention to the nontargetlike pronunciation that causes a communication breakdown. Without such input, learners must hope their own pronunciation accuracy is "close enough," and may continue to (subconsciously?) substitute L1 or IL sounds for L2 sounds that they either do not possess in their IL phonetic inventory in general, or that exist in L2 phonological environments that would prohibit a sound's use according to their L1 or IL rules.

Noticing the "hole" (C. Doughty & Williams, 1998a, 1998b; Swain, 1995, 1998) in one's own IL, however, is even less likely with regard to pronunciation. Noticing the hole refers to recognition of the immediate need for a form not currently in one's own IL, in order to convey an idea in oral or written output. The spontaneous recognition of a missing lexical or structural component often halts output while the learner searches for it, or for an alternative. In contrast, learners rarely become independently aware of the need for a phonological form that they do not know or cannot produce when trying to articulate a thought. Pronunciation is distinct from other areas of L2 learning in that NNSs cannot be aware of the need for a sound unless they have heard it first. Even if they are aware of a "hole" in their phonetic inventory, it will not likely prevent learners from completing the utterance; they will merely substitute their usual IL form for the target form, and continue on with the statement. Thus, it would seem that most noticing in this capacity would pertain to a "gap" rather than a "hole." At best, NNSs may notice phonetic or phonological "holes" upon encountering unique orthographic symbols, diacritic marks, or combinations of the two that differ

8 This does not pertain to the well known 'lisped' pronunciation of the letter 'z' or 'c' (when followed by 'e' or 'i') attributed to many regions of Spain, but rather to the letter 's' as in *supongo* ("I suppose.")

from the L1, and recognize that they do not know what sound to attribute, which could compel them to seek input.

However, there is an additional type of noticing that may be unique to ILPh. It occurs when learners are fully aware perceptually that the sound they are producing is not targetlike, but cannot figure out how to physically modify their articulation to produce the target variant, despite having some metalinguistic information about what they "should do." The above example of the Spanish /s/ can also fall under this category. This situation is particularly difficult, since with lexical or structural holes, an interlocutor could simply provide the model, which the learner could feasibly recognize for what it is and "fill the hole," whereas pronunciation has a potentially confounding neuromuscular obstacle. There is a sense of frustration that is experienced time and again in unsuccessfully trying to form the desired sounds, as if trying to move forward but feeling physically stuck or being held back by some force. Perhaps this awareness would be more accurately described as "noticing the snag." The challenge for the learner, then, is to figure out how to "unhook" himself.

The Need for Phonological Sensitization and Resensitization

"[W]hile several factors predict stabilization, [...] just one factor *sensitivity to input*, is the most likely explanation for fossilization" (Long, 2003). Since learners regularly fail to perceive the communicative value of many L2 sounds, often due to their lack of phonetic salience, much of the facilitation of noticing is ultimately left in the hands of the teacher or researcher. However, since the abandonment of the Audiolingual method, most test-oriented, grammatical, paper-based, or purely communicative instructional approaches have ignored pronunciation on the whole, dismissing it as irrelevant, unnecessary, unteachable, and even socially and culturally inappropriate (Benrabah, 1997; Markham, 1997; Morley, 1991; Pennington, 1998; Pennington & Richards, 1986). Many universities' intensive English programs do not assess oral production as part of diagnostic placement examinations (even if they do offer pronunciation classes), and internationally recognized standardized tests such as the TOEFL only began to include oral skills, including pronunciation, as recently as late 2005. Although potentially well intended, the implication is that learners don't need to pay attention to the intelligibility of their pronunciation, and that virtually any variation of a phonological form is "targetlike enough." Such broad acceptance may enable premature fossilization by encouraging desensitization to the contrasts instead of raising learners' awareness in ways that might promote acquisition thereof. Markham explains the possibility that

> "due to habitual use of attention and production strategies over time for the L1, the speaker '*de-tunes*' the response characteristics of the perceptual and motor systems to new information or commands (e.g. Flege, 1995a; Pisoni, Lively &

> Logan, 1994). The systems can be '*re-tuned*' under certain circumstances" (1997, p. 28; emphasis mine).

It cannot be assumed that learners will be able to "re-tune" their perceptual and motor systems on their own, particularly since "to detect and to produce the subphonemic details of L2 categories [during automatic processing] requires the inhibition of well established routines so that new ones can be established" (Schmidt, 2001). Thus, re-sensitizing learners to notice phonetic contrasts is a necessary precursor to interlanguage restructuring and learning, and requires a change in current approaches to instruction, learning, research and assessment of L2 pronunciation.

Redirecting L2 Instruction and Redefining Learning as Process

Sensitization is a likely necessity, but the question then becomes what it would look like in instruction, research and acquisition. Doughty has identified an explicit link between SLA theory and pedagogy in general, which seems equally applicable to pronunciation as to grammar or vocabulary: she proposes that language instruction should not concentrate on the individual language components, but rather the actual units of processing themselves (Doughty, in press, as cited in Williams, 2005, p. 679). This kind of input processing has been shown to assist learners in acquiring problematic forms (VanPatten, in press, as cited in Williams, 2005, p. 679). Williams (2005) supports this change in instructional intention, suggesting teachers "provide learners with a guided *opportunity* to engage in cognitive processes that are thought to facilitate acquisition of a targeted form" (p. 679, emphasis in original). Thus, researchers and practitioners alike need to re-evaluate their perspective on L2 pronunciation learning, starting with how the concept of *learning* is defined.

The first step is to redefine *learning* on the level of *processing*, rather than on the level of a finite *product* or *outcome.* Prior to determining *what* is taught, it is essential for theoretical and pedagogical inquiry to adopt a new, process-based, learner-centered approach, and explore *whether* and *how* different elements of L2 pronunciation are processed at a given moment.

It is proposed here that in L2 phonology, learning-as-process can potentially be examined in the disparity between typical accuracy and controlled accuracy. As discussed above, intralearner variation is evidence that learners *can* articulate more L2 phonological forms than they typically *do* employ.[9] This is demonstrated almost universally by learners' propensity to produce more targetlike pronunciation on formal word-list read-aloud tasks than in informal interviews, for example. In these situations, the amount of attention paid to language form directly influences the accuracy of the form itself (Hansen, 2004; Major, 1987;

9 Birdsong (2003) calls for longitudinal studies to seek to more systematically distinguish between these two patterns (as cited in Han, 2004, p. 174).

Markham, 1997). Thus, since arguments about critical periods and the likelihood of fossilization (e.g. Scovel, 1969) tend to be based on what subjects *typically* do instead of what they *can* do, it is possible that any claims about constraints on ultimate potential are premature. Instead, if a learner has been found capable of producing an L2 phonological form in more formal task conditions, but does not use the form regularly in casual speech, this form should be viewed as a likely area for development potential via heightened sensitization and attention to the form, since in this situation, confounding psychomotor components unique to pronunciation do not function as potentially impregnable physical barriers to the acquisition of that form. Moreover, since internal auditory and proprioceptive feedback mechanisms are used by speakers to monitor their own speech (Markham, 1997, p. 132), it is arguable that the learner who has demonstrated even occasional targetlike production of a form should be able to use these feedback sources when attending to it, and learning to become more sensitized to the physical contrasts of the more- and less- targetlike variants. Thus, the focus returns to the need to redirect attention and related processes to the contrasting forms.

The question then becomes one of how to identify processing as it occurs. The past three decades of SLA research have indicated that one generally successful approach to identifying process-oriented learning is via online[10] techniques, as they help to distinguish between competence deficits and processing deficits with regard to ultimate attainment in L2 development (Marinis, 2003). Through looking at online protocols, SLA research has learned much about the possible relationship between attention to form and language development, particularly as facilitated by negotiated interaction. Chapter two will consequently explore the research on attention to form and interaction, in order to establish applicability of related constructs and methods to investigation of interlanguage phonological development.

10 *Online* refers to that which is occurring "in the moment," and has nothing to do with the Internet or any other web-based computer technology.

CHAPTER 2

REVIEW OF THE LITERATURE

INTRODUCTION

The investigation of attentional processing is becoming more prevalent in the field of SLA today. One common means of stimulating and observing attentional processing, particularly in an instructional setting, is through task-based interaction that facilitates negotiation of meaning. However, attentional processing research has yet to be extended and applied specifically to the study of L2 phonological development. To this end, this chapter will review the literature that lends evidence to the potential applicability of interactionist approaches to investigating L2 pronunciation development. As such, the chapter is broken into three sections. First, it will begin with a review of the value of interaction and negotiation of meaning for SLA. Subsequently, a discussion of the role of communicative tasks will follow, identifying task conditions that are necessary to stimulate interactional processes. Finally, it will be argued that under these task conditions, two non-native speakers can direct each other's attention to, and help each other modify, non-targetlike phonological forms.

INTERACTION AND NEGOTIATION OF MEANING

Interaction is recognized as a potential context for SLA, particularly as it provides the opportunity to encounter the need to negotiate meaning. According to Long's (e.g., 1996) Interaction Hypothesis (IH), it is very often through interaction that learners' attention is drawn to language forms in ways that will promote the conversion of input to intake as a necessary step in SLA, as described in chapter one in the discussion of Tomlin and Villa's (1994) model. Interaction, whether between a native speaker (NS) and non-native speaker (NNS), or two NNSs, is a condition that is arguably conducive to SLA because it facilitates attention to form. One way is by providing many opportunities for learners to have to negotiate their understanding of or use of a structure. When a non-targetlike or otherwise misunderstood structure causes a momentary breakdown in communication as a result of the NNS's IL being different from the actual target form, interlocutors are forced to temporarily shift the focus of their attention from the overall meaning of the exchange to the code of the language itself (C. Doughty & Williams, 1998b; Long & Robinson, 1998; Williams, 2005).

Although most studies evaluate the effects of interaction on fluency and lexical or grammatical accuracy, R. Ellis (1999a) also states applicability of the IH for research on L2 phonology:

"The revised IH, with its emphasis on the role that interaction plays in stimulating the learners' attention to form, draws heavily on the current models of acquisition that view intake as a primary stage in the acquisitional process. The IH can be used to address all levels of language—pronunciation, lexis, grammar, and discourse" (p. 235).

The current study will potentially be the first to explore specific evidence of such phonological processing during interaction.

Negotiation of meaning in interaction has been defined in various ways. Broadly, it can be viewed as "exchanges between learners and their interlocutors as they attempt to resolve communication breakdowns and to work toward mutual comprehension" (Pica, Holliday, Lewis, & Morgenthaler, 1989). Long further clarified that it included signals to generate "adjustments to linguistic form, conversational structure, message content, or all three, until an acceptable level of understanding is achieved" (1996, p. 418). More specifically, Lyster summarized many other studies' definitions of negotiation as including "various input modifications and interactional moves including semantically contingent feedback such as repetition and reformulation" (2004). It begins when one interlocutor indicates unsuccessful transmission of the other person's prior utterance meaning (Pica, Lincoln-Porter, Paninos, & Linnell, 1996). Ideally, negotiation of meaning that includes modification of utterances of either interlocutor can serve as the link between input, attention and output (Long, 1996). This connection can be made through various means. Most importantly, negotiation of meaning provides learners with *modified comprehensible input*, *feedback* on the accuracy and comprehensibility of their utterances, and an *opportunity to modify their own speech production* (Pica, 1994). These three roles are described in greater detail below, followed by a brief assessment of the applicability of negotiation of meaning centering on phonological forms.

Modified Comprehensible Input

It is generally unquestioned that access to comprehensible input is one of the most essential conditions for SLA. If the input received, whether from a NS or more proficient NNS interlocutor, is just beyond a learner's current interlanguage (IL) level, it will provide opportunities for the learner to notice the gap, as described in chapter one. Pica (1994) found that negotiation facilitated greater comprehension by allowing NNSs to ask open-ended questions, to which NSs responded by "segmenting" (i.e. isolating the problematic word or phrase) or otherwise modifying their utterances, resulting in more comprehensible input. The likelihood of this noticing is increased if the input is modified specifically to meet the needs of the learner. Such interactionally modified input has been shown to be more potentially advantageous than premodified input in promoting SLA: in addition to being more comprehensible to learners than unmodified input in general, interactionally modified input—in contrast to premodified input—provides learners with quantitatively more input overall and more processing time (Ellis, 1999a), as well as greater opportunity for redundancy of input and repetition (Pica et al., 1993).

Corrective Feedback

When a NNS fails to successfully convey a message, the interlocutor will sometimes indicate non-comprehension. This indication, i.e. corrective feedback, is a *signal* (Pica, 1994; Pica et al., 1989) which is intended to alert the NNS to the existence of a nontargetlike structure (or many) that requires adjustment. Although as of yet there is no consensus on the specific value of error correction as a means of monitoring production (Hulstijn & Schmidt, 1994) or of negative evidence on the whole (Gass, 2003), there is ongoing effort and interest in determining what relative value different types of correction might have for certain elements of language development under various conditions (Iwashita, 2003; Lyster, 2004). Studies have discussed the various possible definitions, roles, and functions of negative and positive evidence, negative and positive feedback, and corrective feedback, with somewhat inconsistent terminology. For the purposes of this work, the next sections will attempt to operationalize the notion of corrective feedback and outline some of the key forms of corrective feedback in interaction.

Defining corrective feedback

Corrective feedback is a complex tool that pertains to an interlocutor's response to a NNS's error. Lyster and Ranta (1997) briefly review some of the divergent labels used in related fields such as linguistics, discourse analysis, psychology, SLA and language pedagogy, depending on the relative goal of the research. Some earlier work focused on the identification of "negative evidence" and "negative feedback," rather than "corrective feedback." Gass (2003) explained that negative evidence (NE) primarily provides information pertaining to the unacceptability of a form. Carroll (2001) further classifies NE much more abstractly, as part of a learner's derived conceptual representation. For her, NE is the product of a top-down inferencing process that "involves a systematic comparison...which leads to the conclusion that some property is not part of the grammar of the language" (p. 21). NE can be provided preemptively, as is often done by teachers in a classroom setting, or reactively in interaction, in response to a learner's non-targetlike utterance (Gass, 2003). It is this reaction to a learner's error that requires further distinction.

The interlocutor's response that specifically attends to the unacceptability of the learner's utterance is what is referred to as negative feedback (NFB), and allows for a bottom-up process of comparison in retrospect, from which the learner can "derive positive and [reactive] negative evidence about the second language" (Carroll, 2001, p. 21), where positive evidence (PE) is information about what *is* possible in a language.

Gass further specifies that when NE is reactive, it can be explicit or implicit (2003). If it is explicit, she explains, it will take the form of some sort of overt, deliberate correction. If, however, it is implicit, NE may take the form of a recast (explained in greater detail below), which includes PE via offering a targetlike alternative to the original utterance, or else cause a communication breakdown, potentially requiring negotiation of meaning.

With regard to applicable forms, Carroll (Carroll, 2001) clarifies that NFB can pertain to not only lexical, morphological or syntactic structural choices, but to pronunciation and other components of language as well, as she demonstrates with the following example, in which person-A is L1-English studying German, and person-B is L1-German:

a. A: is it [flanzənkatalɑg]?
b. B: [katalo:g] nicht [katalɑg], we don't have [ɑ]. It's so easy.
c. A: Yes, but is it [flanzənkatalɑg]/ [katalog]
d. B: /[katalo:k] ... yes
e. A: I mean is it plural in this sort of compound or what?
f. B: [pflanzən] yes (Carroll, 2001, p. 22).

She points out that although the learner is seeking grammatical input, the NS interlocutor instead chooses to give feedback on the inaccuracy of her pronunciation, both explicitly regarding her vowel in line (b), and implicitly regarding the need for her to devoice the final consonant in line (d) above.

This study in particular is seeking information about these negotiations and other ways that interlocutors attend to non-targetlike—specifically phonological—form. As such, it almost always addresses reactive statements following learner error (i.e. feedback), and the PE and NE that may be entailed, all of which seem to have an inherently corrective potential function, intentionally or otherwise. This ultimately corresponds to the function on which Lyster and Ranta focus, error correction, in their study on "corrective feedback" as found in "negotiation of form in communicative classrooms" (1997, p. 37). Thus, for the purposes of this study, the term "corrective feedback" (CFB) will be used to subsume these other terms unless otherwise specified.

Types of corrective feedback

It is not just the existence of CFB on the whole, but rather the type of feedback a learner receives that may differentially catalyze restructuring processes and thus potentially influence language development as the learner attempts to utilize the feedback and reformulate the original utterance (Lyster, 2004). CFB types can be distinguished in part by two key features. The first is their relative explicitness, where explicit CFB contains some overt indication of an error in the speaker's previous utterance, but implicit CFB does not contain any such overt sign (Ellis, Loewen, & Erlam, 2006). Skehan proposed that the more consciously aware learners are of the CFB, the more likely it is to facilitate lasting restructuring (as cited in Lyster, 2004). It is for this reason that Ellis, et al. (2006) prefer more explicit forms of CFB, arguing that learners are more likely to become aware of them than of more implicit forms. The second distinguishing feature of CFB types is whether or not they offer a model of the TL form. Both options have potential advantages. On the one hand, CFB that provides the target form offers an ideal opportunity for learners to notice the gap without interrupting the flow of communication (Long, 1996). Yet on the other hand, CFB that does not offer the TL form is more likely to promote negotiation of form (rather than simply negotiation of meaning) by providing the learner with an opportunity to search his own IL for an alternative form, and self-correct (Lyster, 2004; Lyster & Ranta, 1997). Several commonly studied types of CFB moves are identified as follows, particularly with regard to these two features:

1. Recasts

A recast is an implicit form of corrective feedback[11] in which the interlocutor changes one or more nontargetlike components in a NNS's utterance while retaining the original meaning (Long, 1996). Recasts have the potential to "facilitate the encoding of new declarative knowledge" (Lyster, 2004). As demonstrated in Carroll's example above in which the NS identified the need for a word-final devoiced [k], negative feedback is often implicitly provided in the form of a recast, reactively rephrasing the NNS's original utterance in a more targetlike way, thereby not only indicating that the utterance was ill-formed, but also providing positive evidence by modeling what should have been said. In Foster and Ohta's (2005) excerpt below, three L1-English learners of Japanese (referred to as I, J, and E, respectively) discuss homestay families:

I5: Oh. Ee aa kazoku no yoo na (.) Does that work? Depending on family?
Oh. uh uh like a family (.) Does that work? Depending on family?
J6: ah ah ah
E7: Yes.
J8: Yotei? Yote? Kazoku kazoku ni yoote:.
(J attempts to say "Kazoku ni yotte" "depending on the family" but mispronounces the verb)
E9: Kazoku ni yotte.
Depending on the family (correct)
I10: Kazoku ni yotte
Depending on the family (p. 423, original translation and explanation)

11 See Ellis, Loewen and Erlam (2006), however, for a discussion of the more explicit nature of some types of recasts. In this case, however, such *corrective recasts* usually serve as an instructional strategy deliberately employed by teachers, rather than as the more typical meaning-focused negotiation strategy when used by other interlocutors.

Student I seeks input to fill a hole in his interlanguage in line I5, for which student J offers a more accurate but still errant solution, making several phonologically inaccurate attempts to articulate it in line J8, perhaps testing hypotheses (Swain, 1998) for himself (or herself) about how it should sound. In line E9 student E finally recasts J's erroneous utterance, providing the target form which student I immediately incorporates to modify his (or her) own original production, demonstrating uptake, i.e. a reaction to the feedback that somehow demonstrates recognition of the corrective nature of the feedback (Lyster & Ranta, 1997).

Recasting is a commonly employed condition in attentional research, and has been found to trigger noticing under some conditions (C. Doughty & Varela, 1998; Iwashita, 2003; Leeman, 2003; Lyster, 2004; Philp, 2003). There is evidence to show that it can be particularly successful when a preselected form receives regular and/or frequent treatment (Williams, 2005).

2. Explicit Correction

Explicit correction is also similar to a recast in that it directly provides the target form to the learner, but also usually includes a direct alert to the NNS about the error in his speech, such as "You mean," or "You should say" (Lyster & Ranta, 1997). Explicit correction can also encompass a multi-part combination of other feedback types that include both the target form (recast) and either a metalinguistic explanation or other more implicit feedback component. Carroll's above example demonstrates explicit correction in two ways in line (b). The NS first says "[katalo:g] *nicht* (not) [katalɑg]" which begins with a recast of the desired target form, followed by a segmentation of the learner's nontargetlike utterance for contrast, and directly states that it is somehow ill-formed. He then follows with a metalinguistic explanation of the exact nature of the problem element, "we don't have [ɑ]." (Metalinguistic feedback, as an independent category, will be explained below.)

It should be reiterated that, as Lyster (2004) explains, although recasts or explicit correction can be valuable CFB as sources of comprehensible input that provide opportunities to notice the gap and "facilitate the encoding of new declarative knowledge," (p. 406) he does not label them as "negotiation of form" (p. 404). This is because they provide alternative target forms for the learner (Ellis, 1999c; Iwashita, 2003; Lyster & Ranta, 1997) when the listener presumably *understands* the general meaning of the NNS's utterance, and do not require learners to attempt to modify their production. Learners may misinterpret recasts as verification that their message was understood, either ignoring the feedback completely or simply responding "Yes," as in "that's what I said," or "that's what I meant." After explicit correction, learners may simply respond, "Okay." At that point, it is less likely that learners have noticed or otherwise processed the error or target form.

Negotiation moves, in contrast, are generally the result of communication failure when the listener *cannot* understand the meaning of a NNS's utterance due to grammatical, lexical, phonological or other problems (Iwashita, 2003). As such, they are more likely to cognitively engage learners (Lyster, 2004) by directing the learner's attention to the problem form, requiring the learner to search his interlanguage for alternative ways to reformulate his original, erroneous utterance, testing new hypotheses as well. In other words, negotiation moves function as prompts, and "can enhance control over already-internalized forms" (Lyster, 2004) and lead to student generated repair (Lyster & Ranta, 1997). The next four types of corrective feedback, below, are all classified as "negotiation moves."

3. Confirmation Checks

Confirmation checks are also implicit, targetlike reformulations of a NNS's ill-formed utterance, but differ at least partially from a recast in at least two ways. First, confirmation checks are generally used when there is some uncertainty as to the NNS's intended meaning, and thus might not provide the form that the NNS actually needs. Second, confirmation checks use rising intonation to indicate the uncertainty regarding the intended form, implying, "did you mean to say X?" as in the example below:

NNS: this country like bik
NS: big?
NNS: yeah (Pica, 1993, p. 440, as cited in Pica, 1994, p. 514).

As in the previous two categories, this example demonstrates a potential drawback to confirmation checks, which is that by providing a targetlike form, the learner might not recognize their corrective intent, bur rather interpret them as indicating message comprehension (Lyster, 2004).

4. Metalinguistic Feedback

Metalinguistic feedback explicitly indicates that a form is nontargetlike. Such comments may be as simple as "No," or "That's not how you say it." Carroll's L2 German example above illustrates this as the NS explains, "*nicht* (not) [katalɑg]." More informative metalinguistic feedback typically contains metalanguage that points to the nature of the problem, such as "Shouldn't it be in the past tense?" or "Don't forget to pluralize the noun." This is demonstrated in the next line of Carroll's same example: "we don't have [ɑ]." However, metalinguistic feedback by itself does not provide the target form for the learner (Lyster & Ranta, 1997), in contrast to explicit correction, although it is possible that CFB could contain a combination of these two forms.

5. Clarification Requests

Clarification requests are implicit forms of CFB that can indicate a problem in message comprehensibility, a problem in form accuracy, or a problem in both areas simultaneously. Such requests follow learner errors, prompting the learner to try again independently, e.g. "Excuse me?" Although clarification requests do not provide the target form, they may include a segmentation of the error itself to help the learner identify the problem more clearly, e.g. "What do you mean by X?" (Lyster & Ranta, 1997). For example, in the following exchange:

NNS: the windows are crozed
NS: the windows have what?
NNS: closed
NS: crossed? I'm not sure what you're saying there
NNS: windows are closed
NS: oh the windows are closed oh OK sorry (Pica 1992a as cited in Pica, 1994 p. 514)

the NS's first turn is a clarification request. When the learner's second attempt is still unsuccessful, the NS's next utterance segments the problematic phrase, attempting to guess what the NNS had said, and gives a more explicit indication of a communication failure with the illocutionary force of a second clarification request: "I'm not sure what you're saying there." Finally, the learner focuses his articulation enough to intelligibly communicate the key word, "closed." Although there are some examples of TL incorporation here, the necessary target form is not provided as part of the clarification request itself. In line 4, "crossed," though *a* TL form, does not fit the NNS's intended meaning, and the NS's repetition of "closed" in line 6 does not serve to request clarification, but rather indicates comprehension and acceptance of the NNS's independent provision of the required form.

6. Repetition

Repetition is an isolated segmentation by the interlocutor of the erroneous utterance, often with rising intonation to make the problematic form more salient, as in the following example:

St: *Le...le girafe?* [Error-gender]
T3: *Le girafe*? [FB-repetition] (Lyster & Ranta, 1997, p. 48)

Here, the student (St) hesitantly attempts an utterance but errs with regard to the grammatical gender of the noun. The teacher (T3) responds by repeating only the error itself back to the student but with a questioning intonation, as if to rhetorically imply, "are you sure it should be X?" Repetition is included in many other combination forms of corrective feedback such as in Carroll's example above, when the NS interlocutor explained "*nicht* [katalɑg]," repeating the non-targetlike utterance while explicitly indicating that it was problematic. As such combining is typical, only feedback turns that are comprised of repetition alone can be identified as *repetition* itself; repetition combined with other CFB forms is typically classified by the additional component (e.g. metalinguistic feedback), as this is what distinguishes one form from another (Lyster & Ranta, 1997).

Once an interlocutor has provided the NNS with some form of negative feedback on her initial utterance, it often will "push" her to reformulate her own statement in a more targetlike and comprehensible way (Swain, 1985). The potential benefits of such modified, "pushed" output are described in the following section.

Modified/pushed output opportunities

Nearly 25 years ago, the discussion about the potential role of output itself as a requirement for SLA began (Swain, 1985) and has remained a focal issue ever since. One of the most valuable functions of output is that it can "force the learner to move from semantic processing to syntactic processing" (Swain, 1985, p. 249). The potential to stimulate this transition from semantic to syntactic processing in the context of interaction can perhaps be best summarized as follows:

> Negotiating meaning needs to incorporate the notion of being pushed toward delivery of a message that is not only conveyed, but that is conveyed precisely, coherently, and appropriately. Being 'pushed' in output...is a concept parallel to that of the i+1 of comprehensible input. Indeed one might call this the 'comprehensible output' hypothesis. (Swain, 1985, p. 249)

Ultimately, output allows learners to test hypotheses about language use, notice holes in their interlanguage, and potentially restructure their interlanguage upon correcting identified errors (Swain, 1985, 1998). It is this final restructuring process that requires further explanation.

When a NNS's non-targetlike utterance is met with corrective feedback, whether from internal or external sources, the learner may respond to the feedback by attempting to clarify his initial statement. This type of modification is often referred to as *pushed* output (Swain, 1985). As Lightbown explains, "a reformulated utterance from a learner gives some reason to believe that the mismatch between learner utterance and target utterance has been noticed, a step at least toward acquisition" (1998, p. 193, as cited in Smith 2005 p. 39). This pushed output, or modified comprehensible output, may be evidence of uptake, and thus may be a precursor to or evidence of IL restructuring. (For a review of operationalizations of uptake, see Smith, 2005).

Pushed output can result from having received external CFB from an interlocutor, or from the internal realization that one's own utterance was non-targetlike. The high occurrence of self-initiated, self-completed modifications as a normal learning strategy (compared to other-initiated and other-completed modifications) across task and interlocutor (NS vs. NNS) variables in Shehadeh's (1999) study lends strong support to the argument that "learners' output should be given a more *active* role in second language learning" (p. 665, italics in original).

Pushed output can potentially influence two types of acquisition: Internalization of new forms, and increased control over already internalized forms (Swain & Lapkin, 1995).

Sometimes, even without CFB from an interlocutor, the act of producing output can facilitate self-correction, particularly with regard to pronunciation, because the learner has at least two primary internal feedback sources at his disposal: auditory and proprioceptive (Markham, 1997). In other words, the learner has the potential to recognize that his utterance does not sound how he wants it to sound, and to feel that the articulation within his mouth may not have felt how he knows it should have felt. This may be what occurred in the following example:

> "*Dry fruits* ([fru:its])...*fruits* [fru:ts]), *for example, or fresh vegetables...*" (García Mayo, 2005, p. 391, original emphasis).

This may also be evidence that the opportunity for output itself is conducive to noticing and modifying phonological forms. This potential link between noticing, negotiation, and pronunciation is discussed in greater detail in the following section.

Negotiation of Meaning Due to Pronunciation

Like virtually all language components, nontargetlike segmental and prosodic forms used by learners can bring about a breakdown in communication, as demonstrated in several of the CFB and output examples, in various languages, above. Such pronunciation errors may trigger corrective feedback, particularly negotiation moves, leading to modified (phonetic) output. Through these exchanges, interlocutors provide opportunities for NNSs to notice a phonological gap or hole in their IL. This is consistent with R. Ellis' statement about the application of the IH to pronunciation, as delineated on the first page of this chapter.

Task-based Negotiated Interaction

The challenge then becomes how to engage learners in an interaction that would draw their attention to target forms via negotiation. In a typical classroom setting, a logical choice is through targeted communication tasks. This section will identify the most commonly accepted conditions a task should balance for the greatest likelihood of facilitating attentional processes via negotiated interaction. In particular, the need for a balance between communication requirements and target form requirements will be explained. Subsequently, the potential value and feasibility of establishing these task conditions in order to specifically stimulate attention to phonological forms will be demonstrated.

Communication requirements

First and foremost, the primary value of a communicative task is its requirement that learners attend to meaning as an overarching goal of the experience, with their attention being drawn only temporarily to the language form or code, as necessary to address a nontargetlike utterance, most likely due to a perceived breakdown in communication (Long, 1996; Pica et al., 1993; Williams, 2005).

Complementing the meaning-focused nature of the communicative task, Pica et al. (1993) emphasize a mutually required exchange of information between interlocutors in order to facilitate the greatest likelihood of receiving comprehensible input, corrective feedback and modified output opportunities. They specify that as part of this exchange, both interlocutors should be required to request needed information from—and provide needed information to—each other. Additionally, closed-tasks, or tasks with a singular correct outcome, have been shown to be greater contexts for negotiation of meaning because of the need to reach consensus (Pica et al., 1993). Ideally, factually and linguistically accurate exchange of that specific information should be necessary for both parties to meet a common communicative goal and successfully complete the task.

For these reasons, two-way information gap tasks (IGTs) have been identified as being highly likely to facilitate "modified interaction among participants and orient their attention to form, function and meaning" (Pica, Kang, & Sauro, 2006, p. 301). IGTs that require a two-way exchange of essential information to reach the only correct possible outcome increase the likelihood of noticing target language forms. Additionally, well-designed IGTs can draw learners' attention to language forms that are at a developmentally appropriate level yet remain challenging for learners due to their complexity and/or low salience (Pica et al., 2006). (See this article also for a thorough discussion of the contributions of IGTs to interaction research.)

As Shehadeh (1999) explained, "...when successful completion of the task depends primarily on the NNS supplying accurate and comprehensible output...a higher proportion of extended negotiation routines is more likely to occur" (p. 659). When this need for accurate and comprehensible output results in negotiation that centers on the target form, that form incidentally becomes the temporary object of the learner's attention, a condition that is generally recognized as desirable to stimulate processes such as noticing (e.g., C. Doughty &

Williams, 1998b; Ellis, 1999c; Long, 1996; Long & Robinson, 1998; Williams, 2005). In order for such stimulation to occur, there is also the need for interlocutor feedback on the accuracy of the form in question as it pertains to their ability to collaboratively complete the otherwise communicative task (Loschky & Bley-Vroman, 1993).

Target Forms

Once the communicative requirements have been established, and it is likely that learners will attend to various possible language forms at some point in the task, the focus then turns to whether or not such a task can be used to deliberately direct learners' attention to specific target forms. Linguistically targeted communication tasks, or "focused communication tasks" (Williams, 2005), are most valuable as a means of drawing attention to forms that are difficult to learn, often due to their low salience, which otherwise would continue to go unnoticed by the learner. Low salience can be represented in several possible ways, the most common of which are (a) due to low frequency of occurrence, (b) due to low perceptibility, and (c) due to opacity of the relationship between meaning and function (Pica et al., 2006). As the number of phonemes and prosodic patterns is comparatively limited in a given language, there is inevitably ample frequency of their occurrence. Thus, their low salience is most likely due to other low salience features such as their lack of independently held meaning, the lack of perceptible contrast with other L1 or L2 sounds, or the position of the phoneme within the word.

One way in which attention to form can often be stimulated through cooperative tasks is under the condition that successful task completion requires regular exposure to and/or use of target forms that may be inherent in the material (C. Doughty & Williams, 1998b; Pica et al., 1993). The effectiveness of various kinds of communicative tasks may be directly related to the essentialness of the target form to successful communication (Spada, Lightbown, & White, 2005). Loschky and Bley-Vroman have identified three levels of involvement that a particular language form can have in a given task: *task naturalness, task utility* and *task essentialness*, in order of likelihood to facilitate SLA (1993).

Levels of Involvement

According to Loschky and Bley-Vroman's explanation, *task naturalness* simply means that a particular form may occur naturally in the language used to complete a given task, but that the task might just as easily be successfully completed without it. *Task utility* is more potentially facilitative of acquisition because the form is not only natural to the task's performance, but is directly helpful—though still not necessary—to successfully complete the task. It is the final category, *task essentialness*, that is seen as most valuable because the essential form would be absolutely required for the task to be successfully completed.

Loschky and Bley-Vroman clarify that the degree of involvement of a form is not an inherent property of the form itself, but rather relative to the conditions of each unique task. (1993, p. 132). In order to reach this goal, they subsequently explain that it is generally necessary to establish conditions that render the target form essential to the successful performance of the task. In addition to requiring interlocutor feedback on the target form's accuracy, they specify that this may include controlling the rest of the discourse more tightly to increase the likelihood of a form to be required.

Proactive target form selection

If a communicative task is designed with intent to direct learners' attention to specific forms by making accurate use of the form essential to successful task completion, where "essentialness" is not inherent to a form but rather relative to the nature of the task, then it would seem of paramount importance for the researcher or instructor to use extreme care in selecting target forms for a given task. In SLA research, such proactive selection and application of a form for focused attention has become more commonplace (C. Doughty & Williams, 1998b; Williams, 2005). A key consideration in proactive form selection is that learners be developmentally ready to learn a targeted form (Pica et al., 2006). One common approach to finding a developmentally appropriate form is for teachers or researchers to select a form (usually morphosyntactic) having previously observed problems in learners' IL with that construct. Williams refers to this as an IL-based problem (2005, p. 674). A regularly occurring IL-based problem indicates that the learner has a strong communicative need for the form in question, and it may also indicate that the learner is developmentally ready to process, learn, or automatize that particular form. The selected form can then potentially be embedded or otherwise targeted in a focused communication task.

Balancing communication and form requirements on L2 pronunciation tasks

Loschky and Bley-Vroman argue that a key problem with regard to grammar is that grammar tasks don't make the necessary connection between a grammatical form and successful communication, and assert that many information gap tasks "lack specificity in terms of the linguistic focus of instruction" which may result in their lack of regular success as grammar development tools (1993, p. 125). The same can certainly be said for the lack of correlation between phonological form and "successful" communicative task completion. Yet they claim that the principles of task-essentialness of form should be equally as applicable to pronunciation-based communication tasks as to any other language form (1993, p. 157). Nevertheless, most pronunciation textbooks and research tools alike fall short of designing communicative tasks in which phonological forms are even useful, much less essential, to successful task completion. Pronunciation activities tend to be designed to one extreme or the other: to one end, they are often strictly decontextualized, metalinguistic exercises with no greater communicative value, such as word lists to be read aloud or minimal pair drills, the former of which not only lack inherent communicative value, but also lack any interaction requirement or required use of a target form in order to be completed, successfully or otherwise. At the other end, many activities are fully communicative, hyper-contextualized activities, such as open dialogue, which could be (and typically *are*) completed without ever utilizing the target form. Figure 2.1 below summarizes the (im-)balance of communicative value and form essentialness found in some of the most common pedagogical activities (e.g., Beisbier, 1995; Dauer, 1993; Gilbert, 1993; Miller, 2000) and research tools (e.g., Abrahamsson, 2003; Díaz-Campos, 2004; Koren, 1995; Park, 2000; Stokes, 2001) in L2 pronunciation.

This is not to say that these tasks and activities have no inherent value, but simply may not maximize attentional processing opportunities. For example, many textbook pronunciation activities may have instructions that explicitly remind students to monitor for a particular phonological form while talking to a partner, but the lack of task-essentialness of the form itself could result in students' nearly total focus on meaning, ignoring or otherwise forgetting about the intended linguistic target.[12]

Figure 2.1 – Relationship between relative essentialness of form for task completion and overall communicative value of common L2 pronunciation tasks and elicitation tools

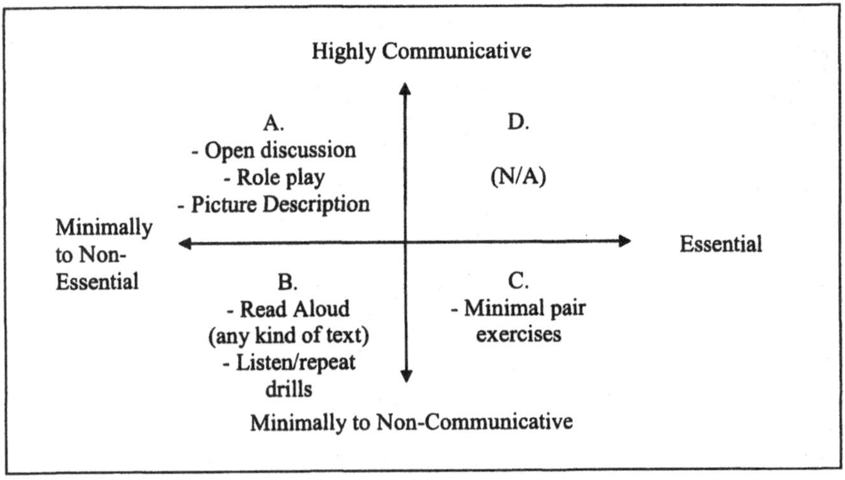

12 This has been my observation with my own students time after time when facilitating many of the more open communicative activities in pronunciation textbooks.

Although language redundancy may make the goal of balancing communicative value and task essentialness a challenge for some phonological forms, it should not be impossible for all of them. The design of a communicative task that makes target phonological forms essential to task completion—and thus fitting in Quadrant D in Figure 2.1 above—will be described in chapter 3.

Task-based Attention to Phonological Form within NNS-NNS Negotiated Interaction (an impossible trifecta?)

Can communicative tasks provide NNSs with opportunities to notice phonological forms? To date, no study has published research data on a task that that specifically targets L2 phonological forms while balancing the aforementioned requirements of communication and form essentialness. (But see Pica (1984) for several types of communicative, targeted pronunciation activities.) However, there is evidence to show that learners' attention can be drawn to phonological forms during other communicative tasks. Mackey, Gass and McDonough (2000) have shown that in *NS-NNS* dyadic interaction in which NSs provided corrective feedback on nontargetlike utterances, learners accurately perceived the intention and target of 60% of the phonologically oriented feedback (which was 41.5% of all episodes), but only 13% of morphosyntactic feedback (which was 47% of all episodes) (p. 483-485). This could indicate that during communicative interaction, learners are even more likely to experience intake regarding phonological forms than morphosyntactic forms overall, despite the propensity of researchers to study the latter.

But what is the potential value of having learners work *together* towards such goals? This issue is far more contentious, and has inspired skepticism from researchers as well as practitioners. The instinctive response many experts from both groups have voiced is, "Why would you want two NNSs to work together on pronunciation? They'll just end up sounding like each other!" The next section will present evidence to debunk this long-standing myth and argue in favor of NNS-NNS dyads working on pronunciation tasks.

NNS-NNS interaction and language learning

Increasing acceptance of the potential value for NNS-NNS interaction in language learning has paralleled the general educational trends of the past several decades, shifting from the teacher-centered classroom to more student-centered, cooperative learning environments. Bruton and Samuda's (1980) ground-breaking study identified that when working with NNS peers, child learners not only recognized errors and made modifications to their own output, but that they also noticed errors in their partners' speech, and attempted to draw the speakers' attention to the errors by asking a clarification question or offering an alternative phrase, with only one recorded instance of an interlocutor mis-correcting an initially targetlike utterance. Gass & Varonis also found that learners not only repair non-targetlike forms in each other's utterances, but that they will incorporate repaired forms into subsequent speech (1989).

Since then there have been many studies that have contributed to a general recognition of the potential for language learning via NNS-NNS dyadic interaction (e.g., Bruton & Samuda, 1980; Gass & Varonis, 1989; Long, 1996; Long & Porter, 1985; Pica et al., 1996; Varonis & Gass, 1985). Pica, et al. noted that NNSs "have been found helpful in providing each other with feedback signals and responses that contain modified output" (2006, p. 303). Not only do they provide each other with these signals and responses, but also often engage in more negotiated interaction with each other than with NS interlocutors. This is in part because NNSs offer less CFB containing target forms than NSs do (Long & Porter, 1985; Pica et al., 1996), and "often relinquished control of discourse" on tasks when working with NS interlocutors instead of modifying output or signaling non-comprehension (Pica et al., 1989, p. 78). Additionally, the NNS-NNS environment is less threatening than when working with a NS interlocutor, which may encourage learners to request clarification or otherwise indicate nonunderstanding (Gass & Varonis, 1985; Iwashita, 2003). As further evidence, Shehadeh (1999) found that NNS-NNS dyads completing a picture dictation task offered more other-initiated negotiations leading to modified output than were found in NS-NNS dyads on similar tasks. Indeed, this exemplifies a trend showing that NNS-NNS combinations tend to stimulate more negotiated interaction than NS-NNS or NS-NS overall (e.g., Bruton & Samuda, 1980; Long, 1996; Long & Porter, 1985; Pica et al., 1996). These findings reveal many previously unrecognized language learning opportunities, as Gass & Varonis (1989) succinctly explain: "It is clear that [systematic investigation into the nature or function of repairs in NNS-NNS dyads] is an important forum for gaining input, since, in general, learners spend a great deal of time conversing with other NNSs" (p. 76). This is certainly the case in both second- and foreign-language classrooms alike.

NNS-NNS interaction and L2 pronunciation

How far do these findings extend? Is it possible for the NNS-NNS condition to facilitate attention specifically to phonological form? L2 Pronunciation curriculum designers in general seem to work under the assumption that it is possible, as textbooks have also followed these educational trends, incorporating more and more pairwork into their lessons (e.g., Beisbier, 1995; Dauer, 1993; Gilbert, 1993; Miller, 2000; Reed & Michaud, 2005), despite the aforementioned skepticism pertaining to the logic of NNS-NNS combinations for learning pronunciation. Is it simply a marketing ploy following general educational preferences for student-centered classrooms, or is there genuine theoretical and pedagogical value in such a design? It will be argued here that there is substantial evidence to indicate that the NNS-NNS condition is neither futile nor counterproductive but rather facilitative of L2 pronunciation development.

In contrast to the fear that "they'll just sound like each other," Jenkins found that particularly when two NNS interlocutors are of different L1 backgrounds, they will indeed accommodate their pronunciation by modifying it away from their respective L1s and towards a more targetlike form for mutual intelligibility (2000). This is consistent with Long and Porter's (1985) findings about ideal NNS dyadic combinations for language development potential, specifically, that two NNSs of different L1 backgrounds working together are more likely to engage in negotiated interaction than will two NNSs of the same L1 working together.

As further evidence, Bitchener (2004) found that NNS-NNS dyads collaborating on spot-the-difference and decision-making tasks signaled pronunciation problems in 17.3% of the negotiated episodes. He speculates that the number may have been even higher if fewer of the dyads had been NNSs with a shared L1 (eight of the 15). This also supports Jenkins' (2000) and Long and Porter's (1985) findings. Yet despite the mix of divergent or shared L1s, 69.6% of pronunciation triggers were modified overall, and more of the NNS interlocutors' signals were modified (e.g. recasts) than unmodified, thereby allowing the original speaker to accept and employ the provided model when reformulating their output. This is in contrast to signals in response to lexical or grammatical problems, which were more frequently unmodified than modified. Yet on the one-week and 12-week delayed task repetitions, 93.7% and 87.5% of the negotiated and modified pronunciation items were retained, respectively, compared to 61% and 54.2% of vocabulary items, and 85.7% and 71.4% of grammatical items, respectively. This evidence demonstrates that on linguistically untargeted communicative tasks, learners can not only identify each other's non-targetlike pronunciation and draw each other's attention to it, but also provide, comprehend, and incorporate modifications in pushed utterances.

Additionally, Garcia Mayo (2005) found that not only will NNSs correct each other, but that they are able to self-correct pronunciation when working together, and that in NNS-NNS dyads, five out of 55 repairs were pronunciation-based, as in the following (aforementioned) example:

> "*Dry fruits* ([fru:its])...*fruits* [fru:ts]), *for example, or fresh vegetables...*" (p. 391; original emphasis).

Although the interlocutor did not provide any CFB, the NNS-NNS condition still provided the opportunity for a learner to produce output, and subsequently notice and accurately modify phonological forms, which could have happened regardless of the interlocutor's L1. This corroborates Shehadeh's finding that more repairs were self-initiated than other-initiated, regardless of whether or not the interlocutor was a native speaker (1999). In this situation, the non-native ability of the interlocutor becomes a non-issue, and may be further evidence that the mere act of producing output itself is facilitative of noticing phonological forms, perhaps moving not from semantic to *syntactic* analysis, as per the original comprehensible output hypothesis (Swain, 1985), but rather moving by the same process from semantic to *phonological* analysis.

NNS-NNS dyads pose an interesting challenge for researchers: discerning at what point an utterance is considered to be (modified) comprehensible input, vs. (modified) comprehensible output. The same utterance can have both functions, because "[i]n exchanges between learners, one learner's modified output is another's comprehensible input" (Ellis, 1999b). For the purposes of this study, what is important is simply whether learners attend to phonological forms and modify their pronunciation, regardless of which function it serves at a given moment. Hence, "modified pronunciation" will be used interchangeably with "pushed output," "modified (comprehensible) output" or "modified (comprehensible) input," as necessary and situationally appropriate, unless otherwise specified.

NNS-NNS interaction on phonologically targeted communication tasks

To date, it does not appear that a strategically designed, linguistically targeted, and communicatively structured pronunciation task has been attempted, so there is little to no empirical evidence that such an approach would not stimulate online attentional and learning processes. Thus, it is time to formally put some of the varying beliefs to the test, and design a communicative task in which particular L2 phonological forms are made to be task essential, in attempt to elicit NNS-NNS negotiation of form via modified interaction, demonstrating evidence of possible online learning-as-process of L2 pronunciation. The following research questions guided this investigation:

RESEARCH QUESTIONS

1. When working together on interactive pronunciation tasks, can NNSs draw each other's attention to targeted phonological forms in ways generally understood to facilitate SLA?
   1a. Do they provide each other with corrective feedback on the target form?
   1b. Do they modify their production of the target form?

2. If NNSs do provide each other with corrective feedback that focuses on the target form, are there specific ways in which they do so?

3. If NNSs do modify their target form production, do the modifications result in more targetlike pronunciation?

Chapter three will describe the methodology that was used to investigate attention to phonological form in NNS-NNS negotiations during communicative pronunciation tasks.

CHAPTER 3

METHODOLOGY

INTRODUCTION

This chapter identifies the setting, participants, activities (pre-task activity and main task) and administration of the study that examined how NNSs attend to phonological form during task-based negotiated interaction. An outlined explanation of the rationale for various aspects of the task design, administration and data collection procedures, and coding scheme are included. As this was a process-oriented study, there was no pre-test or post-test administered. Finally, data analysis procedures are described.

SETTING

This study took place at the Intensive English Program (IEP, pseudonym), for international students, at a large, private university in the summer of 2005. The students come from a variety of linguistic and cultural backgrounds, though the majority of the participants are from east Asia. The program identifies eight proficiency levels: levels 100-400 are known as elementary, levels 500-700 are intermediate, and level 800 is advanced. Students are initially placed into a level as a result of their placement examination scores upon arrival at the university. The tests administered are the listening comprehension and structure sections of the *Comprehensive English Language Test*, published by McGraw-Hill, and a written composition test which is an in-house tool used to elicit a basic writing sample. The listening comprehension and structure components are standardized, multiple-choice format, and the writing component is a written prompt to which students can freely respond. It is important to recognize that there is no speaking component, so *pronunciation is not a factor in determining students' proficiency levels*. After each eight-week session, students generally progress to the next level. All students in the IEP are asked to sign a basic consent form upon enrolling in the program, allowing their work to be observed for research purposes.

While each intermediate level has its own multi-skill "core" class requirements, there are other more specific intermediate electives that can be taken by students at level 500, 600 or 700, and these classes usually have a mix of students from all three levels. Elective classes meet four days per week for 65 minutes each time. One such class will be called Pronunciation Development (PD), which is the setting for this study.

Once a week, each PD class had a regularly-scheduled meeting at the multi-media language laboratory ("the lab") instead of in their usual classroom. All students had become familiar with the lab equipment and general procedures prior to the data collection session for this study. In the lab, each student sat at a station equipped with—among other things—a Sony Student Cassette Deck (model ER-9030) player/recorder and Sony (HS-90) headsets. The quality of headphones and microphones on the headsets was sufficient to allow very high and low vocal frequencies to be clearly transmitted, thus phonemes such as [s], [f] and [θ] were clearly distinguishable. The hardware on the teacher console utilized a Sony (LLC9000/Robotel M-160) system, from which the students could be digitally paired.

PARTICIPANTS

In this study, three PD classes ($n^a = 16$; $n^b = 16$; $n^c = 15$) participated. The PD classes were chosen for several reasons. As the course is an elective, motivation to improve pronunciation and participate fully in activities should be equally high for all students. More importantly, intermediate, or at least post-beginner learners have been identified as benefiting more from significant negotiated interaction than beginning or otherwise unready students, particularly for certain key or targeted structures (Iwashita, 2003; Pica, 1994). Moreover, it is important to remember that (a) degree of L2 phonological proficiency does not tend to correlate to degree of grammatical competency, oral fluency, or overall perceived L2 proficiency, as mentioned in chapter one; (b) pronunciation abilities do not play any role in determining a student's placement in the IEP; and (c) PD classes are comprised of a mix of students from all three intermediate levels. Thus, it can be presumed that the combination of students in any in-tact PD classroom will, by default, have a random mix of pronunciation abilities. Table 3.1 below shows a breakdown of the L1 distribution and gender composition of each class.

TARGET FORM SELECTION

As mentioned in chapter 2, linguistically targeted communication tasks can be a valuable means of drawing learners' attention to forms of low salience. In this case, researchers or teachers select an emergent form they believe their students to be ready to learn, having observed IL problems with that form previously. This section will describe various factors leading to the proactive selection of *theta* (/θ/) as the target form for this study.

Table 3.1: Distribution of L1 and gender in PD classes

L1	Class A, n=16 (5 male, 11 female)	Class B, n=16 (7 male, 9 female)	Class C, n=15 (5 male, 10 female)
Japanese	2	9	5
Korean	9	4	2
Chinese (Taiwan)	2	3	5
Spanish	3	0	2
Russian & Chinese[13]	0	0	1

Loschky and Bley-Vroman explain that there are two identifications that need to be made to select a target form for a pedagogic task: identification of the problematic contrast, and of the potential cause of the problem (1993). For the purposes of this study, the segmental form *theta* was chosen as the target form, as it meets both criteria. First, /θ/ is one of the English phonemes not found in the native languages of most of the participants[14], and typically replaced with other contrasting English phonemes such as /s/, /t/ or /f/. It is commonly found to be difficult for adult L2 learners to discern aurally, and rarely articulated in free conversation, despite the fact that most NNSs can physically produce it orally when asked to do so. Second, L1 transfer is generally accepted as the primary influence on foreign accent, as explained in chapter one, thereby affecting which phonemes are substituted. Thus, Loschky and Bley-Vroman's two criteria have been met.

Informal observation by participating teachers confirmed that none of the students had fully automatized targetlike use of *theta* 100% of the time in obligatory contexts, (and most virtually never used it in free speech at all.) There are several common phonemes that NNSs will substitute when speaking in English. Typically, the segments [s] and [t] are substituted. However, occasionally [f] is substituted by some learners, depending on the L1 dialect or position and phonetic environment of the *theta* within the word. Less frequently, /θ/ is omitted completely—such as in the word-final position by many L1 speakers of Vietnamese. Table 3.2 provides a breakdown of typical substitutions for the *theta* by L1 group.

13 This student was actually born in Turkey, but relocated internationally several times in childhood, adolescence and adulthood. Thus although Turkish was technically his "first" language, he considered his "primary" and dominant languages to be Russian and Chinese.

14 Although it is found in Castilian Spanish, and three of the participants were from Spain, the orthographic referents for /θ/ in that dialect would be a 'z' or 'c' (if followed by 'e' or 'i'.) Despite its inclusion in the L1 phonological inventory, Castilian-Spanish speakers tend to associate the spelling of 'th' in English words with the phoneme /t/ (if unvoiced; otherwise /d/) and make phonetic substitutions accordingly.

Table 3.2 – Typical phonemic substitutions for theta by L1 group

/s/	/t/	/f/
Czech German Hebrew Continental French Japanese	Spanish Hindi Hungarian Italian Canadian French Portuguese Swedish Korean Farsi Vietnamese Turkish	Brazilian Portuguese+
French* Chinese* Slovak*⁺ Polish* Arabic* Russian* Dutch* French*	French* Chinese* Slovak*⁺ Polish* Arabic* Russian* Dutch* French*	French* Chinese* Slovak*⁺
* These speakers may substitute multiple phonemes, depending on the dialect of the L1, phonemic environment or position within the word. ⁺ These data have been observed on multiple occasions by the researcher personally while working with an L1-Slovak student at the time of this study.		
Table data (except for Slovak) are compiled from Archibald, 1998; Avery & Ehrlich, 1992; Swan & Smith, 1987.		

It is also worth noting that some of these commonly substituted phonemes are parallel to substitutions used by L1 speakers of nonstandard varieties of English as well as child L1 development of standard English. For example, in a typical New York regional variety, [t] will replace /θ/, and Cockney speakers will often use [f] (Avery & Ehrlich, 1992), as will many speakers of African-American Vernacular English (AAVE) (Rickford, 1996). Additionally, in child L1 development, English-L1 children often substitute [f] for /θ/ in words such as *thumb*, resulting in [fʌm] (Finegan, 1999, p. 561), or [t], changing *think* to *tink* (Bowen, 1998). Thus, the substitution of these phonemes by L2 learners is a natural phenomenon that may be part of a developmental sequence that is phylogenetically and ontogenetically (Major, 2001) related to language contact and dialect variation, and L1 developmental stages, respectively.

MATERIALS DESIGN

This section will articulate the rationale behind the design of two process-oriented activities, a pre-task activity and the main two-way information gap task, intended to direct learners' attention to the target form *theta* by stimulating negotiated interaction with peer NNS interlocutors. As this was a process-oriented study, ultimate attainment was not the focus of the research and is beyond the scope of this investigation; thus, no pre-test or post-test was used. Instead, the primary distinction in the activities lies in the attentional demands placed on students as a result of task complexity (Robinson, 2001b) which will be described in greater detail in subsequent sections.

Loschky and Bley-Vroman (1993) explain that "the goal in a grammar-based production task is to focus the learner's processing capacities on the meaningful function of a specific structure" (p. 140), and that "communicative structure-based production tasks will be most valuable as 'practice' activities to develop automatization of a specified structure" (Loschky & Bley-Vroman, 1993, p. 141). With a pronunciation-based application of this assertion in mind, the goals of the main information gap task were to promote negotiation to see whether learners were able to draw each other's attention to the form *theta*, and help each other produce and perceive target-like articulation thereof as they carried out the task as possible evidence of a step in the process of automatization.

However, prior to looking for evidence of automatization, Bitchener explained that with regard to learning pronunciation through incidental negotiation, "researchers need to...distinguish between items that have momentarily been forgotten and those that were not known prior to their exposure during negotiation sequences" (2004, p. 94). Unfortunately, the reality may be that it is not such a clear-cut distinction with L2 phonology, as learners may "know" an "item," and indeed *think* that they *are* using it, but not actually articulate it in a targetlike way during production. Duff (1993) also warned that elicited data from one task type will not show the range of learner ability. Thus, if they do not employ a particular phonological form, is it because they are not attending to it, or because (for whatever reason) at the moment, they physically cannot produce it? To address this question, a pre-task activity was designed as prerequisite to participation in the main task.

The pre-task activity

The pre-task activity was comparatively formal[15], with intent to generate simple, decontextualized utterances containing samples of learners' production of the target form. It has low linguistic and cognitive complexity with a single task demand (Robinson & Lim, 1993 as cited in Robinson, 2001), following patterns not unlike the minimal-pair exercises in the students' textbooks, but modified to facilitate greater two-way communication between NNSs. It was not only intended to orient learners' attention to the target form (c.f. Tomlin & Villa, 1994) but to show what learners optimally *can* produce when able to maximally focus attentional resources on the target. In other words, it allowed participants to demonstrate their level of acquisition of theta at the least automatized/most conscious level, and thus demonstrate whether they possess the neuromuscular capacity to perceive and produce the target form under the least and most demanding word positions, i.e. in word-initial and word-final (and medial) placements, respectively.

If the pre-task activity data showed that a participant was unable to articulate the target form successfully (or, hypothetically, in contrast, if he had a profound frontal lisp, which would result in the opposite problem, substituting /θ/ for [s] nearly every time) on the pre-task, there were several possible considerations regarding how to treat that person's subsequent participation data on the main task. On the one hand, although neuromuscular impediments may have prevented them from articulating the target form, regardless of the amount of noticing and attentional processes they undergo, it was not necessary to discount their exchanges in overall analysis. This problem of articulation would not necessarily prevent their perception from becoming more attuned to the distinction by the end of the task, and they would still be able to help direct their partners' attention to the target form and help push their partners to modify their pronunciation in turn. It would also be valuable to identify what alternative negotiation strategies they employed to get their partners to understand which form they were intending to say at these moments. The coding of such data will be discussed at the end of this chapter.

The pre-task activity also served to orient student attention to the target form in hopes of increasing the possibility of detection thereof (Tomlin & Villa, 1994) prior to engaging in the more challenging main task. The decontextualized and cognitively- and linguistically undemanding pre-task activity was performed prior to the highly contextualized and more cognitively- and linguistically- demanding main task, which placed other attentional demands on the participants. This sequence is intended to promote the greatest possible fluency and accuracy (Robinson, 2001b).

15 "Formal" here is intended in the linguistic sense, not the sociolinguistic register sense, as distinguished in chapter one.

In this pre-task activity (see figure 3.1), participants each receive identical lists of double sets of adjacency pairs in which the only difference between each set of initial sentences is a minimal pair word. This format is similar to exercises found in the students' pronunciation textbooks and frequently used in their class, so it should have been comfortably familiar to participants. Minimal pair words were included in which the /θ/ is contrasted with /s/, /t/ and /f/, and in which the target phoneme contrasts are found in the word-initial, -medial, and -final positions, with the contrasting segments textually enhanced (underlined) to orient the participants to the target feature. Tomlin & Villa (1994) view input enhancement as a means of increasing salience of critical form distinctions to raise awareness and ultimately improve the likelihood of their detection (p. 199).

Figure 3.1: Samples of sets of adjacency pairs in the pre-task

	Sentence	***Response***
i.	*a) That child is very mousey.*	*a) I wonder why he's so shy.*
	b) That child is very mouthy.	*b) I wonder why he's so rude.*
ii.	*a) We have thought about that a lot.*	*a) But we haven't come up with a decision yet.*
	b) We have fought about that a lot.	*b) But we haven't come up with a compromise yet.*
iii.	*a) I only have a pair of threes.*	*a) I am not good at playing poker.*
	b) I only have a pair of trees.	*b) I am not good at gardening.*

From each numbered pair of sentences, one partner read either *sentence-a* or *sentence-b* aloud. The other partner listened to determine which sentence was said, and read aloud the corresponding response phrase, where *sentence-a* always corresponds to *response-a*, and *sentence-b* always corresponds to *response-b*. This is to avoid the possibility of students giving the wrong answer due to misunderstanding the meaning of the sentence or response. (See Appendix A for the full text of the pre-task.) If the correct response was given, students went on to the next set on the list and changed roles. If the wrong response was given, interlocutors were supposed to address the problem before moving on. It was ultimately left to the participants to determine what was sufficient.

Upon completion of the pre-task activity, participants went on to engage each other in the main task. The main task was a cognitively and linguistically demanding map task, requiring participants to attempt more unscripted speech and process more information in order to complete it successfully.

The map task

The main task employed a specially designed map, and required interlocutors to give each other directions along streets on the map. Several researchers have used maps to elicit various elements of discourse. For example, Robinson and Lim (1993) used multiple map tasks to look at relative fluency and accuracy in interaction when under different task demands. In one condition, the route between two locations was provided, thus requiring one participant to simply articulate the given route to his interlocutor (single task demand). In the other condition, no route was provided, thus the first participant had to both select the route for himself and subsequently articulate it to his interlocutor (multiple task demand.) Robinson asserts that task complexity affects negotiation and interaction by proportionally increasing the need for interlocutors to confirm and clarify points, which thereby "confirms the relationship between communicative demand and cognitive demand" (2001b, p. 49). Thus, in the map task for this study, multiple task demands and greater complexity were intended to provide for optimal negotiation (Robinson, 2001), while still keeping the majority of negotiation episodes relating to the central phonemic item of focus. The specially designed map was the object of discussion in a two-way information gap task, centered on the [θ] phonemic distinction, and required two-way communication with exchange of independently held information for successful completion.

For this task, student pairs received identical street maps of an imaginary city, "New Philadelphia" (see Appendix B.) Maps were designed with the streets in a grid format in which parallel street pairs have minimal-pair names. For example, Booth Road runs parallel to, and one block over from, Boot Road. One corner is numbered at each intersection, with the intersection at the top left corner of the page receiving the number 1, and all other intersections receiving numbers systematically in order, working towards the bottom right corner of the page so that they are easy to find. At the top of the map are two lists (A and B) of four (4) locations each, such as "City Hall" and "the Art Museum." Each person was assigned List A or List B, and was instructed to independently assign a different numbered corner to each of the four respective locations.

One participant (the "receiver") then began by asking her partner for directions from any intersection of her choice to one of the locations on her partner's list, e.g.: "How can I get to City Hall from the intersection of Boot Road and High Path Road" (compared to Booth Road and High Pass Road, or a different combination thereof as possible.) The interlocutor then gave compass-based directions, such as, "From Boot Road and High Path Road, go east to Theme Park Drive, then turn south and go to Mossy Hill Street. City Hall is on the northeast corner. What number is it?" The receiver responded with the number that corresponded with the point at which she arrived. If she was correct, the partners switched roles for the next item on the other person's list. If she was not correct, her partner had to make a second attempt to re-direct her from start to finish again. Dyads were told that they could interact as much as necessary to clearly give and receive directions.

Participants also received an instruction sheet (see Appendix B) along with the map. This page included suggestions for basic direction-giving commands in case this would prove to be an unnecessarily challenging component for some. The language used to give directions is fairly routinized in English, but customs and real-world application and experience can be problematic if students have never been in the specified situation. For example, if learners have never purchased international airline tickets over the telephone or given directions in English, they will not know what topics or gambits are relevant (Gorsuch, 2001) for such an occasion. The instruction sheet also delineated restrictions for what could *not* be included in the directions, most notably any form of numbers. Thus, for example, students were not allowed to give the number of the intersection from which they wanted to begin or at which their partner needed to turn, nor could they indicate the number of blocks to go in any direction. All directions had to go by street names and compass directions (north, south, east and west) or relative directional words (right, left, up and down) alone, in order to force partners to rely on the clarity of their pronunciation to effectively guide each other to the desired end points. These instructions emerged from the understanding that "in order to make structural accuracy essential to accurate communication of meaning, the designer of the task must exert a great deal of *control* over the discourse in the task" (Loschky & Bley-Vroman, 1993, p. 140).

It is important to recognize that the potential negotiations would almost always begin from the receiver's initial request for directions, since every intersection is near three others that sound almost exactly like it, distinguishable only by the target phoneme. For example, the intersection of High Path Road and Boot Road is very close to the intersections of a) High Path Road and Booth Road, b) High Pass Road and Boot Road, and c) High Pass Road and Booth Road. Thus, the person giving directions inevitably asked for some confirmation or clarification that he was beginning to direct the receiver from the correct starting point. Once the starting location had been established, he needed to provide the instructions, and then it was the receiver who needed clarification at any or every street corner to which she was directed. Hence, at different stages of the same set of directions to a single destination, both interlocutors were required to provide and request uniquely held information, and both had the opportunity to request and provide clarification in order to reach a mutual endpoint. Also, since participants arbitrarily assigned intersection numbers to the destinations, and arbitrarily chose starting points for each round, the same pattern should never have been repeated, and participants were not be able to anticipate how far they would have to "walk." This provided learners with ample opportunities to provide and receive comprehensible input, modified output and corrective feedback (Pica et al., 1993).

However, the map task also provided ample opportunity for repetition of information, which is valuable to SLA for several reasons. Since giving directions includes rather formulaic language routines, it facilitates repetition and thereby limits the amount of new information that must be processed overall. Repetition is also important because recycling items in the process of resolving communication breakdown should raise the likelihood that learners will notice key forms, as the increased frequency can raise their saliency (Long, 1996). Additionally, Bygate establishes the value of task repetition and familiarity, as content mastery allows learners to focus attentional resources on linguistic features to promote accuracy (as cited in Bitchener, 2004). Loschky and Bley-Vroman add that learners need multiple opportunities to move from noticing the problem to finding the cause, restructuring hypotheses and finally automatizing (1993, p. 153-154). Thus, it was also important to design a task that allowed for as much recycling as possible, in order to facilitate the increased salience and subsequent noticing, and restructuring, particularly for linguistically targeted tasks. The map task allows for this condition, in that participants had to negotiate their way along the same streets up to eight times, which should have allowed them to orally and aurally distinguish the street names more easily with each subsequent repetition.

PROCEDURES

Preparation

The two instructors (one is the researcher, who taught both classes A and B) agreed to teach the segment /θ/ during the first weeks of the session, using the usual class textbook *Targeting Pronunciation* from Houghton Mifflin. Lessons on phonemes include (but are not limited to) explicit instruction on the physical properties of articulation for /θ/, minimal-pair drills and exercises contrasting /θ/ to other phonemes such as /s/, /t/ and /f/, and practice dialogues incorporating the target sound. This guarantees that all students had, at the very least, the same amount of formal, explicit instruction and practice opportunity focusing on the target form immediately prior to data collection, and with approximately the same interval of time between this instruction and the data collection period.

In week five, after each teacher had sufficient time to introduce and reinforce the target form, each teacher took her class to the lab for their weekly multi-media activities focusing on the target form. The pre-task activity and map task served as the class materials for the day.

Dyad assignment

Dyads were deliberately assigned, rather than randomly, for several reasons. Primarily, it has been understood that the greatest potential for SLA is facilitated in NNS-NNS dyads when interlocutors are of different L1s and different proficiency levels, as established in chapter two. Based on the size and demographic breakdown of the classes, random assignment would not likely maximize these conditions.

Therefore, as attendance permitted, dyads were established in which interlocutors were first and foremost of differing L1 backgrounds. The research has emphasized the need for paired NNSs to be of different L1s as the most ideal condition for promoting SLA in dyadic interaction (Bitchener, 2004; Griggs, 2005; Jenkins, 2000; Long, 1996; Long & Porter, 1985). Griggs (2005) explains that if NNS-NNS dyads share the same L1 and/or same proficiency level, they may resort to L1 use, particularly if there is a minimal gap between their respective abilities and knowledge. This is of particular importance with regard to pronunciation, since the L1 is the strongest influence on L2 phonological development, as explained in chapter one, so interlocutors of different L1s may be more likely to notice non-targetlike pronunciation in each other's speech. As such, this assignment attempted to control for L1 combinations as a first priority. Proficiency, however, should not have been a problem in this case, since pronunciation ability has no correlation to assigned proficiency level in the IEP, and should not have influenced overall communication ability since the language of the tasks is rather tightly controlled, as explained above.

Data collection

Data collection occurred in one hour-long session for each of the three classes, during which participants completed the pre-task orientation activity followed by the map task.

After dyads were formed, each dyad was assigned to a console and instructed to put on headsets with earphones and microphones through which interlocutors would talk to each other. The headphones also helped block out most other ambient sounds. Additionally, dyads were told to sit with their backs to each other so that they could not see each other's face and were thereby forced to rely strictly on oral communication through the headsets. This arrangement was intended to "prevent any paralinguistic or nonlinguistic interference" (Shehadeh, 1999, p. 633). Paralinguistic and nonlinguistic cues are referred to here as "interference" because they are compensatory, and lessen the need for accurate target language production or perception. As the pre-task activity and map task were designed to lead participants to rely on accurate articulation and perception of target phonemes and orally negotiate their way through problems thereof, the ability to rely on hand gestures or lip-reading, for example, would have defeated the purpose. A cassette recorder was a part of each station, and each dyad was given one high-bias cassette to record their assignments for the day.

Once dyads were settled at their stations, the teacher passed out the pre-task activity sheets. Instructions were read aloud by the researcher as participants read along on their own copies. The teacher then modeled two examples with one volunteer to demonstrate the rules and allowed for participants to ask questions in order to clarify rules and procedures. The teacher then instructed the group to press the *record* button on the cassette decks and perform the pre-task activity, stopping the cassette when they had finished.

Subsequently, the map and map task instruction sheets were distributed. Instructions were read aloud and one example set of directions was given in the same way as during the pre-task. However, prior to the model set, all street names were read aloud by the teacher, and repeated by the participants. This served two purposes. First, if vocabulary was unknown, students would not have been able to discern if the words contained new or salient information (Gorsuch, 2001). For this study, this also meant learners may not have known how to pronounce the rest of the key words, regardless of the target sound, and may have allowed orthography to negatively influence their pronunciation, as explained in chapter one. For example, when contrasting "Coral Wreath Lane" and "Coral Reef Lane," learners might incorrectly assign sound to the otherwise silent /w/ or /a/ in *wreath.* This could help their partner to identify the intended word of the minimal pair, whether or not they accurately pronounce the distinguishing word-final consonants /f/ or /θ/. Thus, all words were modeled by the instructor prior to the task, to allow students to hear, repeat, and make any notes for themselves to facilitate the accuracy of their own pronunciation of the target words during the task itself. (Ultimately, this did not prevent all such errors, but likely reduced the frequency thereof.)

As with the pre-task, once all questions were answered, participants were instructed to press the *record* button and begin the task, and stop the cassette upon completion.

Data Analysis Procedures

Transcription

Once the tasks were completed and had been recorded on the cassettes, the interactions were transcribed. Transcription reflected non-targetlike pronunciation in cases involving the target form *theta*, or in cases where the pronunciation may have caused misunderstanding and/or a breakdown in communication. IPA symbols were only occasionally used, particularly when a schwa (ə) was epenthesized in noteworthy places, or generic orthographic conventions would not clearly convey the nature of a problem. Additionally, *italics* were used to convey vocal emphasis via raised pitch/intonation, and colons (:) were used to indicate gemination, or elongated sounds. A question mark (?) represents a word- or phrase-final rise in intonation in a way that sounds like a question, but has no bearing on the syntactic structure of the utterance. A comma (,) represents a brief, mid-utterance pause, whereas a period (.) indicates falling intonation and pause that indicates the end of a declarative statement-type utterance. Ellipses (…) represent a longer pause than a period, often indicating someone trailing off mid-utterance before continuing the point, and lasts approximately one or two seconds. Finally, numbers in parentheses indicated the number of seconds of silence during longer pauses between utterances, generally two seconds or longer, rounded to the nearest approximate second. Transcription assistants were trained by the researcher, who did most of the transcription, and who subsequently verified all transcription clarity and accuracy herself, and accepts responsibility for any inaccuracies therein.

Coding

One additional person worked with the researcher to code the task transcriptions. The researcher trained the other coder personally. Both independently coded each transcript using the operationalized categories defined by the researcher. The researcher then compared the results, and non-matching codes (including lines in which only one coder had assigned a code at all) were addressed in two steps. First, if it seemed obvious that a difference was due to simple oversight or "slip of the hand" (Fromkin, 1980) on the researcher's side, she amended her code. (See examples in the CFB section, below, particularly regarding the blatant PE/PI distinction.) Or, if it seemed equally obvious that there was the same kind of oversight or "slip" on the part of the other coder, then, without explanation, the researcher first provided a list of transcript line numbers for the second coder to blindly review, i.e. to recode without looking at her own original code choice. This resolved approximately 75% of discrepancies, upon comparison of the new responses. Although it could be argued that asking the coder to revisit certain lines could have led her to assume a need to change her response and adjust accordingly, two considerations should have prevented any significant effect on validity. First, the request for the "blind" review would prevent her from remembering her own original code assignment (or lack thereof,) so if she reassigned the same code twice, it would likely confirm her conviction of its accuracy, though this was rarely the case. Second, as the nature of the discrepancy was not provided in the review request, and there were many possible combinations of codes (including no code) available, it was not possible for her to predict the researcher's desired response.

Second, any remaining discrepancies were then discussed. If it became obvious that a difference was still due to oversight (e.g. having missed contextual data to verify a modification—see below) or "slip," the mutually agreed-upon code was assigned. If a difference in interpretation was not immediately and easily resolved at that point, it was left as a point of disagreement.

After intensive training using two transcripts, this system was used to code a representative sample of five more transcripts (23.8% of the total), and inter-coder agreement was established at 91.07% reliability.[16] At this degree of agreement, the reliability score was generalized to the remaining transcripts and the researcher coded the rest independently. Transcriptions were coded for two key features, in accordance with the focus of the research questions: corrective feedback and target-form modification, both of which are operationalized below.

Corrective Feedback (CFB)

First, corrective feedback (CFB) is identified as a signal in which one person indicates a breakdown in communication (Pica et al., 1989). This breakdown could be due to her own non-comprehension, at which point the CFB would signal a need for additional comprehensible input. Alternatively, the CFB could indicate that one person notices an error in her interlocutor's speech and sees a need to address and correct the problem. As CFB indicates a lack of clarity of form or meaning, it draws attention to some part of the previous utterance. For the purposes of this study, CFB was classified on two broad levels: implicitness vs. explicitness of the negotiation move, and implicitness vs. explicitness with regard to the existence of the phonological form in question, whether the target form, *theta,* or its minimal pair alternative. Table 3.3 below shows samples of the resulting four types of CFB classifications identified.

Prolonged silence or other fillers marked by prolonged duration or flat low pitches, for example, could also be viewed in certain contexts as implicit negotiation moves, e.g.

1. S1: Turn right on High Pass Road.
2. S2: Which?
3. S1: High Path.
4. S2: U::::::h... (2)
5. S1. Path, Path.

16 It should be noted that entire transcriptions were searched by both coders for evidence of attention to form, rather than taking a short excerpt of recordings for transcription and coding (e.g. Shehadeh, 1999; Foster & Ohta, 2005), limiting analysis to learner responses to a limited number of key NS prompts (Mackey, Gass & McDonough, 2000) or a finite number of pre-selected utterances for coding or rating, as is often done for testing intelligibility (Munro, Derwing et al., 2006). Thus, a possible alternative reliability measurement could have included all of the lines that both coders agreed – on first pass – did *not* contain any outward evidence of attention to form, i.e. received a "no-code" code. If that measure had been used, the number of turns (lines) coded with agreement would have been in the thousands, with disagreements remaining in low double-digits, thereby raising the inter-coder agreement level to 98 or 99%.

If communication had been successful, S2 would have been able to respond in such a way as to promote additional exchange of information in line 4. Thus, in addition to his first utterance, 'Which?', and his second comment, 'U::::::h," S2's silence serves as CFB (category = PI-NI) and implies a breakdown in communication. S1 infers it as such and recognizes the need to provide additional input, which she does in line 5.

Table 3.3 – Examples of four corrective feedback types

	Phonologically Explicit (PE)	Phonologically Implicit (PI)
Explicit Negotiation (NE)	*I said 'Path,' not 'Pass.'*	*Can you say it again?*
Implicit Negotiation (NI)	*'Pass' or 'Path'?*	*Excuse me?*

It should be noted that the PE/PI distinction is essentially a black-and-white distinction, i.e. either a street name keyword with the target form (or its alternative) is included in the utterance (PE), or no such word is included (PI). This made recognition of the aforementioned "slip of the hand" easily identifiable in coding and analysis.

The NE/NI distinction is more complicated. This is not to be confused with explicit vs. implicit *correction*, which is commonly discussed in the field of SLA, and which was described in chapter 2. Rather, it is the explicitness of the negotiation move itself as a means of directing one's interlocutor's attention to form. A classification of NE includes one or more of five possible components. First, an "explicit negotiation" move can contain *metalanguage* such as spelling or description of tongue placement. Second, it can contain *task-based* language, such as, "Which street?" Third, it can contain an *overt negation* of an *error* such as "No," or "Not (X)." The fourth type would be a word or phrase that *heralds*, prefaces, or otherwise points to the word in question, such as "Did you say (X)?" or "I told you it was (x)." Finally, a code of NE could include a *direct request* for input of some sort, e.g. "Once more?" or "Could you repeat that, please?" If one or more of these units is visible, regardless of the role of the person who uttered it, it was marked as NE. If none of these units is visible, but the utterance still functions as CFB, as was the case in line 4 of the previous example above, it was marked as NI by default.

Target-form modification

The second major interaction move analyzed in the transcripts pertained to whether and how NNSs modified the target form. Several factors needed to be considered when operationalizing "modification" of the target form for this task. Ultimately, the participants were not simply learning to produce a phoneme accurately, although this is certainly one form of "more-targetlike" modification. Rather, they were learning to *control for target-like use.* This kind of control means targetlike production *in obligatory contexts*, and in correlation, learning to control against over-suppliance in non-obligatory contexts (Pica, 1988).

For example, as the task provides binary choices, either option could be "correct" depending on the intent of the speaker. In such a case, a participant might say "turn right on North Man's Alley" when he actually meant "Norse Man's Alley." If it became apparent that the non-theta-inclusive street name was indeed intended, and the participant did manage to change from "North" to "Norse," it was coded as a more-targetlike modification, demonstrating control of the form by knowing when it should *not* be present, and being able to clearly articulate the contextual alternative.

In addition, true control of the target form entails not only skills of production, but also perception. Thus, some modifications will be on the part of the listener, rather than the original speaker. For example, in the following exchange:

1. S1: Turn right on Norse Man's Alley.
2. S2: North Man's Alley?
3. S1: No, Norse.
4. S2: Oh, Norse.
5. S1: Yeah.

it does not appear that the problem lies in either person's inability to accurately produce [s] or [θ]. Instead, the listener (S2) misunderstood which he had heard, and upon receiving CFB (specifically PE, NE/overt error negation) in the third line, realized his mistake and changed options. Hence, S2's modification was not in attempt to reformulate the same word, but to demonstrate control via aural ability to distinguish between the two similar options, and would consequently be coded as a "more-targetlike modification" as well. This would also be the case if the above example were reversed, with regard to "Norse" vs. "North," if S1 had originally said "North" and S2 misperceived it as "Norse."

In contrast, modifications were coded as "less-targetlike" if, provided the intended form (whether the theta-inclusive word or its minimal pair alternative) is identifiable from the context of the exchange, a participant is (at least somewhat) targetlike in perception and/or production of the obligatory form, but then produces a subsequent utterance demonstrating a shift that is less accurate. E.g.:

1. S1: Go to <u>Three</u> Town Avenue.
2. S2: Mhm.
3. S1: In <u>Sree</u> Town Avenue turn left.

In such a case, "Sree" is not a viable alternative for either road name, and thus assuming it is clear from the context that S1 was referring to "Three Town Avenue," the modification from [θri:] to [sri:] is clearly less targetlike.

Finally, it is also important to remember that modification can occur not only upon being pushed for clarification through CFB from their interlocutors, but also upon recognition of one's own error. As discussed in chapter two, NNSs have the potential to self-correct upon recognizing their own errors through auditory or proprioceptive feedback, without receiving any CFB from their interlocutors. As a result, there is the potential for the speaker to make a non-targetlike utterance, realize it immediately, and modify her pronunciation, before her interlocutor has a chance to signal a problem, e.g.:

S1: Turn right on *Nors*—ah, *North* Man's Alley.
S2: Okay.

Additional considerations

The NNS-NNS nature of the interaction requires some additional qualification herein. There are three key issues that need to be addressed. First, since minimal pairs are embedded throughout the map, it was not always immediately clear if a speaker had mispronounced a target form or not. It was only upon analysis of the negotiation routine that surrounds it that this distinction could be made. For example, if a speaker said, "Go to High Pass Road," it was impossible to know out of context if he truly meant to say "Pass," or if he actually had intended to say "Path," since both were viable options. E.g.:

S1: Next, walk north until you find High [pas] Road.
S2: High *Path* or *Pass*?
S1: Oh, ah, *Path, Path.*
S2: Path, okay, I got it.
S1: So, at High Path Road, turn east...

Contextual cues to indicate intent could include spelling the word, indicating the intersection number (which would be "breaking a rule" for the task, technically,) or going from one alternative to the other along the route, e.g. starting at North Man's Alley and moving east *to* Norse Man's Alley.

Second, also because both interlocutors are NNSs, it is possible that the speaker's utterance is perfectly targetlike, but a misunderstanding may be caused by a listener's inability to perceive the contrasts easily. Thus, CFB may not necessarily indicate a non-targetlike utterance. Again, this will only become clear upon analysis of the context of the exchange. Once the nature of the problem has been identified, i.e. non-targetlike production or difficulties with perception, it can be further determined if the nature of the exchange serves the purpose of pushing the speaker to produce modified comprehensible output, or of providing the hearer with interactionally-modified comprehensible input, respectively. This latter opportunity is demonstrated in the following example:

S1: Next, walk north until you find High Path Road.
S2: High *Path* or *Pass*?
S1: *Path, Path.*
S2: Path, okay, I got it.
S1: So, at High Path Road, turn east...

As a result of these concerns, modifications were only coded as more- or less-targetlike if it could be determined from the context which word was intended. For example, at the end of a chosen route, the intersection number reported would confirm which street names were used, and thus which phonemes were obligatory. Or, if a speaker produced an utterance that contained a non-targetlike articulation of the target form that is *not* similar to the minimal-pair alternative, as in the above example in which the speaker pronounced "Three" as [sri:], this can also serve as confirmation for which word was intended. If it was not possible to reasonably verify which street was intended, the exchange was considered ambiguous and not included in the analysis.

Third, as mentioned above in the description of the purpose of the pre-task activity, it was possible that a participant may have been completely physically unable to produce the sound [θ], or conversely, had some form of lisp that made [s] difficult to accurately produce. At that point, it was likely that no amount of negotiation in the course of the pre-task activity or main task would have been able to push the learner toward a more targetlike production of /θ/ in obligatory contexts. In such a situation, it would still be worthwhile to analyze the student's modification strategies, but more importantly, it was of value to look at the CFB strategies his interlocutor employed as necessary. The reverse roles were no less valid or valuable: to analyze the CFB strategies of the participant with the speech impediment, or the modification efforts of his interlocutor.

Ultimately, the employment of the coding scheme sought evidence pertaining to whether and how NNSs draw each other's attention to phonological forms. Preferences for various types of CFB were identified, along with the potential for learners to facilitate each other's modification towards a more accurate control over the perception and production of L2 target forms. The results of this analysis are reported in Chapter 4.

CHAPTER 4

RESULTS

INTRODUCTION

This chapter presents the analysis of participants' negotiation of the target form *theta* (/θ/) when working together on communicative pronunciation tasks. Findings reflect data that answer the research questions established in chapter 2. To reiterate, these questions were:

RQ 1. When working together on communicative pronunciation tasks, do NNSs draw each other's attention to a targeted phonological form in ways generally understood to facilitate SLA? I.e.:
- 1a: Do they provide each other with corrective feedback on the target form?
- 1b: Do they modify their production of the target form?

RQ 2. If NNSs do provide each other with feedback that focus on the target form, are there specific ways in which they do so?

RQ 3. If NNSs do modify their target form production, do the modifications result in more targetlike pronunciation?

PRE-TASK MINIMAL-PAIR ACTIVITY FINDINGS

Results of the pre-task activity confirmed that all participants possessed the neuromuscular capability to, at least sometimes, perceive and produce the target form, and successfully distinguish it from the forms /s/, /t/ and /f/, which are often mistakenly substituted for /θ/ by non-native speakers of English. However, it was also determined that six participants did demonstrate non-standard variations on /s/, minimizing the strident properties possibly by changing articulatory features from alveolar to post-dental, or from apical to coronal. Several of these participants showed signs of a frontal lisp, consistently substituting a clear [θ] in place of /s/ in at least some or most obligatory conditions for [s]. This was confirmed by a phonologist in the University of Pennsylvania's Linguistics department, who was otherwise unconnected to this study. Ultimately, it was often challenging for the hearer – whether interlocutor, transcriber or coder – to discern which minimal pair word was being uttered under these conditions. These deviations from the standard were noticeable on many words throughout the interaction, not just on the minimal pair words. The differences were less noticeable and easily overlooked in non-minimal-pair words as the context made the intended meaning recoverable. Nevertheless, what was most important was to verify that all participants were indeed able to produce the *theta*, and this conclusion was reached. The issue of the lisp will be further addressed at the end of chapter 5.

Map Task Results

Of the total 161 destinations to which participants randomly assigned intersection numbers, comprised of 322 street names (two streets per intersection of each destination,) 151 destination streets (46.9%) contained the target form *theta*; the rest contained the minimal pair alternative. This proportion seems reasonable, as exactly 50% of the street options included *theta*, and the other 50% were equally divided between alternative forms /s/, /t/ and /f/ (as explained in chapter 3, and visible on the map in Appendix ___), and participants randomly assigned intersection numbers to their destination place names prior to studying the map.

The following tables show the breakdown of corrective feedback (CFB) moves and target-form modifications, as confirmed by two coders, for each dyad's performance on the Map Task. As described in chapter 3, two broad categories were applied to qualify CFB moves. The first is whether a move was phonologically explicit (PE) or implicit (PI), i.e. whether it explicitly contained the target form or contrast form in the street name, or not, respectively. The second is whether the utterance contained a discourse element that would explicitly mark the negotiation (NE) effort as requesting or providing CFB, or if no such explicit negotiation move was present (NI). Table 1 below shows the total number of moves for each of the four possible combinations.

It can be seen that dyads 5 and 17 had the fewest CFB moves (18) of all dyads that completed all eight task items. Of the 18 total moves, dyad 5 had ten PE-NI moves, one PI-NI, three PE-NE, and four PI-NE moves. In contrast, dyad 17 required the highest number of CFB moves, 65, to complete the entire task. Of those, 42 were classified as PE-NI, one was PI-NI, 16 were identified as PE-NE, and the final six were PI-NE.

It is noteworthy that of the 559 total CFB moves identified, the vast majority (74.4%) fell under the category of PENI. As these moves typically were confirmation checks of sorts, containing little if anything more than the street name in question, e.g. "High Pass?", they were ultimately the most efficient form of CFB, successfully identifying the problematic element and nothing else. Overall, phonologically explicit CFB was greatly favored over CFB that did not contain a target form word (or portion thereof), with a PE total of 88.0%.

Table 4.1: Total Corrective Feedback Moves by Major Category

DYAD*	PE-NI	PI-NI	PE-NE	PI-NE	Dyad Total
1	13	3	2	3	21
2	6	2	5	2	15
3**	17	1	3	2	23
5	10	1	3	4	18
6	21	1	1	2	25
7	40	0	2	1	43
8	23	1	10	12	46
9	38	0	7	3	48
11**	21	0	2	3	26
12	28	0	0	3	31
13	21	3	2	10	36
17	11	1	4	2	18
18	26	2	2	1	31
19	22	1	5	1	29
20**	13	0	8	0	21
21	42	1	16	6	65
22	31	0	0	1	32
23	22	0	0	1	23
24	50	0	10	2	62
25	31	1	6	5	43
26	37	0	4	7	48
TOTAL	416	10	76	57	559
%	74.4%	1.8%	13.6%	10.2%	100.0%

* The numbering system corresponds to the number on the cassette each dyad initially used to record their task. Cassette #10 was corrupted; cassettes #4 and 14-16 were not utilized. There were 21 usable recordings.

** Dyad 3 only completed seven of the 8 total task items, dyad 11 only completed six, and dyad 20 only completed four.

The existence of an explicit negotiation marker seemed less necessary, as only 23.8% of all CFB moves were identified as NE. Thus, it is arguable that learners felt that being explicit with regard to the target form was more communicatively valuable than being explicit in marking their efforts at negotiation.

SUB-CATEGORIES OF EXPLICIT NEGOTIATION (NE) MOVES

As outlined in chapter 3, an explicit negotiation move would be identified as containing at least one of five different types of utterances: (1) metalanguage; (2) task-based language; (3) "heralding," (i.e. linguistically prefacing an utterance); (4) overt negation, or (5) a direct request. Table 4.2 shows the breakdown of NE utterances according to these sub-categories:

Table 4.2 - Breakdown of Explicit Negotiation Move Types

Dyad	MetaLx	Task	Herald	Ovt Neg	Request	Dyad Total
1	0	3	1	0	1	5
2	0	5	0	1	2	8
3	0	1	0	2	3	6
5	0	1	2	2	3	8
6	1	1	1	0	0	3
7	0	1	0	1	1	3
8	0	7	4	4	5	20
9	3	3	2	1	2	11
11	0	3	0	1	1	5
12	0	3	0	0	0	3
13	0	5	0	2	5	12
17	0	2	3	0	4	9
18	0	1	1	1	0	3
19	0	2	4	0	2	8
20	0	2	2	3	1	8
21	0	13	7	3	4	27
22	0	1	0	0	0	1
23	0	1	0	0	0	1
24	1	7	1	3	1	13
25	0	5	3	0	3	11
26	0	8	1	1	3	13
Total	5	75	32	25	41	178
%	2.8%	42.1%	18.0%	14.0%	23.0%	100.0%

From table 4.2, it can be seen that of the 178 total NE utterances, participants used fewer metalinguistic utterances (5 tokens, or 2.8%) than any other type of NE strategy. In contrast, task-based language was the most utilized strategy, with 75 tokens, or 42.1% of the total NE moves. Heralding, overt negation and direct requests each accounted for 32, 25 and 41 tokens, or 18.0%, 14.0% and 23.0%, respectively. Examples tokens of each of the NE types are as follow.

Metalinguistic

Metalinguistic feedback includes any description of, or reference to the language itself. E.g.:

Dyad 6, line 141: "Simple." (i.e. "the one that is easy to say")

Dyad 9, line 194: "Yeah, eh, ah, it's not 'T' 'H' sound." (naming the letters)

Dyad 24, line 299: "[…] This street is pronounce is, Truth Alley."

Task-Based

Task-based feedback includes any utterance that has a direct reference to a description of the map, directions, or other items directly borrowed from the task itself. E.g.:

Dyad 3, line 188: "Can you repeat the first word of the street?" (also includes heralding; see below)

Dyad 5, line 216: "Coral what?" (i.e. "Coral *Reef*" or "Coral Wreath.")

Dyad 17, line 71: "Uh, could you repeat where you started to walk?"

Heralding

Heralding includes any utterance that frames or prefaces the target in question, e.g.:

Dyad 1, line 54: "You say me, eh, Think Street and Free Town Avenue?"

Dyad 18, line 35: Nor, uh, uh. I catched uh uh words of North Man's Alley."

Dyad 25, line 53: "I, I talk um Mo-mo-mossy."

Overt Negation

Overt negation includes any utterance that uses "no," or "not" to explicitly recognize an error, e.g.:

Dyad 1, line 180: "No, Faithful."

Dyad 5, line 102: "Tic, not, not, not, not, "Th:::ick. Ticket, Ticket."

Dyad 20, line 117: "Not Mossy!"

Direct Request

A direct request includes any utterance that announces the need for confirmation, clarification, or other assistance, e.g.:

Dyad 1, line 101: "Uh, can you tell me, again?"

Dyad 3, line 75: "Fee, Fear? One more, fear."

Dyad 8, line 126: "[...] on... Booth Road, right? (2) This is right?"

CORRECTIVE FEEDBACK: OTHER FINDINGS

In addition to the PE/PI and NE/NI distinctions discussed above, it was clear that there were several other discourse features that were used by participants as strategic means to draw each other's attention to the phonological form in question. As these were additional findings, and not part of the original operationalized categories (though ultimately adding another layer of quality to them), intercoder reliability was not established; only the researcher identified these patterns. These strategies included: (1) juxtaposing the minimal pair options for easier contrast, (2) gemination (i.e. lengthening the form,) (3) pausing around the target-form word (and sometimes in the middle of the word, if the target form was medially positioned,) (4) rising intonation on the target-form word, (5) increasing the volume of the target-form word, (6) segmentation (i.e. repeating the target form in isolation, or the syllable that contains it), and (7) schwa-epenthesis. Table 4.3 below shows the distribution of these strategies.

Pausing and intonation were the most frequently employed strategies, often occurring as a set pair. Segmentation occurred the least frequently. It is worth noting that these numbers only reflect findings from the map task recordings, but that even during the simple pre-task minimal pair activity, these strategies were evident, though to a lesser degree.

Table 4.3 – Corrective Feedback, additional strategies

Dyad	Juxt	Gem	Pause	Inton	Vol	Seg	ə	Dyad Tot
1	0	0	17	4	0	0	0	21
2	2	6	7	9	5	0	0	29
3	6	2	6	9	0	0	0	23
5	3	4	21	12	1	1	0	42
6	3	0	5	4	2	0	4	18
7	2	6	7	6	0	1	7	29
8	3	7	6	7	0	0	0	23
9	11	14	11	4	1	1	0	42
11	0	6	10	5	0	1	1	23
12	0	13	20	12	1	0	6	52
13	5	9	9	5	4	0	0	32
17	5	3	10	1	1	1	0	21
18	1	6	11	8	5	2	0	33
19	7	5	10	4	4	0	0	30
20	5	0	0	1	0	0	0	6
21	2	9	15	3	0	0	7	36
22	2	4	19	5	0	0	0	30
23	1	2	8	11	5	1	2	30
24	3	8	13	6	0	2	3	35
25	5	9	27	6	0	0	0	47
26	6	3	2	12	0	0	0	23
Total	72	116	234	134	29	10	30	625
%	11.5%	18.6%	37.4%	21.4%	4.6%	1.6%	4.8%	100.0%

One point here warrants clarification. The epenthetic schwa is distinct from L1-influenced epenthesis. Typically, L1-influenced epenthesis occurred early in the task, or early in a negotiation, and negotiations resulted in modifications that eliminated the epenthesis, making the articulated word more targetlike overall, regardless of whether or not there was any modification to the target form itself. In contrast, strategic epenthesis was identifiable in several ways. Rather than being eliminated as the routines continued, participants often accurately articulated the word- or syllable-final *theta* or alternate form without trouble, i.e. without habitually adding schwa, but later in a routine *added* the schwa in order to make the form in question more salient by creating a new syllable with the problematic form in the onset position. In this case, the newly formed syllable was often stressed via one or more of the additional strategies listed above, to emphasize the deliberate nature of the move. The following excerpt from Dyad 6 illustrates this point:

49.	SuJin:	And, you have to go west?
50.	HeeOon:	Uhuh
51.	SuJin:	until North man's alley?
52.	HeeOon:	North man's uhuh
	[	]
53.	SuJin:	North Man's Alley?
54.	HeeOon:	Uhuh.
	(20 turns)	
75.	SuJin:	Yeah. (2) *Northə*, Man's Alley.
76.	HeeOon:	O::h, okay.
77.	Both:	(Laugh)
78.	HeeOon:	North.
79.	SuJin:	North, Northə Man's Alley.

It can be seen that both interlocutors produced the target form in coda position without trouble in lines 51, 52 and 53, despite the fact that they both spoke Korean as their L1, which does not allow [+ continuant] syllable codas. However, as some confusion occurred later, SuJin chose to emphasize her intended word choice via three measures in line 75: schwa-epenthesis, rising intonation (indicated by italics), and an added pause after "north," allowing HeeOon time to identify and process the contrast. She repeats the strategic schwa use in line 79 as a final confirmation move.

Modification

Throughout the map task, all participants made many modifications demonstrating their relative articulatory control of the target form and its contrasts. However, because participants chose their own start and end points as well as the route between them, at many points it was impossible to verify the speakers' intent, regardless of how clearly they seemed to be articulating one form or the other. This is because both forms were viable options, and occasionally it also became clear that their intended street name did not match what their interlocutors (and transcribers and coders) understood them to be saying. For example, it could be apparent to all listeners that the speaker uttered "Mossy," but if the destination point was at intersection 56 (Mothy Hill Street and Boot Road) it would be evident that either all listeners were misperceiving the utterance, or that the speaker lacked articulatory control (and, it often seemed, lacked awareness of his own inaccuracy.) Thus, the only modifications that are formally included in the analysis are ones that could be contextually verified, as explained in chapter 3.

Verification was possible in several ways. A common one was simply waiting for disclosure of the destination's intersection number, which confirmed two intended street names. Metalinguistic information, such as spelling, was another. Occasionally, directions given would move the listener *from* one street *to* its minimal pair street, which also verified both. Other task-based verification included telling a partner to go as far as possible in a given direction before turning, indirectly indicating it was the last possible street available, geographically. One participant also found a way to "beat the system," so to speak, by leading his interlocutor on a zig-zag pattern through the streets, hitting both streets in a pair whenever possible, which also allowed for easy verification of both. L1-influenced error also was viewed as evidence of intent, e.g. in Dyad 2, Alicia (L1 = Spanish) gave the following instructions:

14. Alicia: until High Path Road?
15. Ul-Sik: Uhuh.
16. Alicia: In High Pat Road you need turn right? [...]

Her utterance in line 16 included "Pat," though the only two options on the map were High <u>Pass</u> Road and High <u>Path</u> Road. As Spanish does allow /s/ in the coda position, "Pass" would not likely have caused problems. However, L1-Spanish learners of English do often substitute [t] for /θ/, as explained in chapter 3. Thus, these issues provide sufficient evidence to code the utterance of "Pat" in line 16 as (-), or a less-targetlike modification.

The final tally of more-targetlike (+) and less-targetlike (-) modifications, as defined in chapter 3, for verifiable street names, is in table 4.4 below.

Dyad 7 was the only pair with no modifications on *verifiable* streets, although both interlocutors did seem to make modifications from time to time in street names that were not verifiable. Dyad 26 seemed to have the greatest challenge with the task, modifying their articulation of verifiable street names a total of 46 times, almost equally in more- and less-targetlike ways. However, the overall total shows a ratio of nearly 2(+):1(-), indicating that there were almost twice as many more-targetlike modifications audible to all listeners (including interlocutors, transcribers and coders) than less-targetlike modifications.

Table 4.4 – Verifiable Modifications

Dyad	(+)	(-)	Dyad Total
1	4	1	5
2	5	1	6
3	3	1	4
5	7	2	9
6	1	1	2
7	0	0	0
8	12	7	19
9	8	3	11
11	1	0	1
12	3	0	3
13	3	1	4
17	9	2	11
18	4	1	5
19	3	1	4
20	4	1	5
21	6	3	9
22	3	0	3
23	3	5	8
24	11	9	20
25	7	4	11
26	24	22	46
Total	121	65	186
%	65.1%	34.9%	100.0%

Summary of Results

In sum, it can be seen that NNSs can and do draw each other's attention to targeted phonological forms through CFB and modification. The CFB can be phonologically explicit or implicit, as can the nature of the negotiation move itself. Additional strategic characteristics of the CFB were also discovered. It similarly became clear that learners do modify their production of the target form and its contrast forms in ways that demonstrate greater accuracy and control over the articulation and perception of the contrasts. Further discussion of these findings can be found in chapter 5.

CHAPTER 5

DISCUSSION

INTRODUCTION

Do second language learners have the ability to acquire the phonological systems of additional languages? If so, are the same processes and conditions identified by SLA research as facilitative of L2 morphosyntactic or lexical development also likely to promote L2 phonological development? Can pedagogic materials be developed through which learners can help each other attend to L2 phonological forms and improve their accuracy and control of those forms? These are some of the fundamental questions that motivated this study. A map task was designed and implemented to seek answers to these questions. It established conditions that SLA research has argued to be facilitative of L2 development in general: it was inherently communicative in nature while holding target form accuracy as essential to successful task completion, in effort to promote attention to a phonological target form through negotiated interaction, including corrective feedback and modified production of the target form, *theta*. But could the pairing of non-native speakers (NNSs) as interlocutors on this task actually help to advance these processes, or would such a condition be futile, or even counterproductive? Rather than helping each other to attain a more targetlike pronunciation, would two NNSs indeed appropriate each other's nontargetlike phonetic production, and in the end, "just end up sounding like each other"?

Analysis of the data provided abundant evidence that pedagogic tasks can be developed through which NNSs can successfully work together to improve their pronunciation. Not only did the learners demonstrate a variety of strategies to draw each other's attention to the target form, *theta*, but they regularly helped each other improve the accuracy of their production as well as their listening comprehension. A deeper analysis of the following excerpt will provide initial support for these claims.

95. Peng[17]: Uhhh, ecuse me. How do I get to, Liberty Bell?
96. Hiroko: Um.
97. Peng: from the ([fr^ŋlə]) intersetion of u::::h... F, F, Fay, Fate, Fatefall, fall, fall, Fatefall, Way,
98. Hiroko: Um-hmm.
99. Peng: anda the...Thru::ce, Thru::ce Alley. Truce Al,
100. Hiroko: Tru::ce Al, Alley? or Tru:th, Alley?

17 All names are pseudonyms that should accurately reflect the gender and L1 of the speaker.

101. Peng: A::h, thu, *thu*, uh, oh sorry. Thr, thr, thruce, chu, chuth, truth, uh truth, Truth Alley, Chruth Alley, Truth Al,
102. Hiroko: Anda Fate,ful, ([feit^h, fʊl]) Way?
103. Peng: Uhh, Fateful Way, yea, Faitthful ([feitθfʊl]) Way.
104. Hiroko: Fait::thful ([feit←::θfʊl])Way?
105. Peng: Uh, fate ([feit^h]), fate, fate, fut, Fateful Way.
[ ]
106. Hiroko: Fate? Okay.
107. Hiroko: And Truth::, Alley?
108. Peng: Yes. Ezactly.
109. Hiroko: Okay.
110. Peng: Truth Alley anda Fatful Way.

In this exchange, Hiroko and Peng successfully demonstrate many explicit and implicit variations on corrective feedback, self- and other-initiated modification of *theta*, and other unanticipated strategies for drawing each other's attention to the target form. For example, there is evidence of corrective feedback in lines 100, 102, 104 and 107, and ample self- and other-initiated modified production and hypothesis testing (Swain, 1998) in lines 97, 99, 101 and 105. As described in chapter 4, the negotiation move in the feedback is implicit, but phonologically explicit, in the form of a clarification request in line 100, as well as in the confirmation checks in line 102, 104 and 107. Additional strategies employed to increase the salience of the form in question are juxtaposition of the two alternatives (line 100), syllable-level segmentation (97, 105 and 106), post-target pausing (100, 102 and 107), and gemination (107). It is also important to recognize that by the end of the negotiation routine, Peng , an L1-Chinese male, and Hiroko, an L1-Japanese female, have reached consensus on the intended forms, modifying their production towards more targetlike accuracy. These modifications demonstrate greater control over perceiving and producing the target form in an obligatory context (Truth Alley), as well as recognizing a context in which it is *not* required (Fateful Way).

The rest of this chapter will explore the patterns identified above as well as in the rest of the findings reported in chapter 4, and discuss implications they may hold for researchers and practitioners alike in the field of SLA in general, and in particular, regarding the acquisition of L2 phonology.

Communication breakdown: Speaker-based vs. Hearer-based Errors

The study of processes and conditions that arise in NNS-NNS interaction has long been of interest and concern to researchers. Especially challenging therein is the study of corrective feedback and modification. First, questions arise in identifying the directionality of the corrective feedback that NNSs provided each other and the relative necessity of their target-form modification. This challenge is due to the nature of NNS-NNS interaction: if a listener does not understand a speaker's utterance, is it because of a deficiency in the listener's perception ability, or was the utterance truly nontargetlike? Thus, if one NNS does not understand the other's utterance, it is difficult for researchers to determine whether this is due to a deficiency in perception, i.e. a hearer-based error, or a lack of accuracy in production, i.e. a speaker-based error. The following excerpt from Dyad 6 demonstrates a hearer-based error:

135. SuJin: and Mossy Hill Street.
136. Park: Mothy?
137. SuJin: Mo, Mossy. Sy.
138. Park: u::h...
139. SuJin: Mossy.
140. Park: Mosthy? Mothy?
141. SuJin: Simple. (Laughs)
142. Park: Ah.

To deconstruct what has occurred here, a line-by-line analysis is valuable. As revealed in this excerpt, SuJin provided a targetlike, non-theta street name in line 135, which Park did not hear correctly, as shown by his erroneous confirmation check in line 136. SuJin then provided Park with additional corrective feedback in line 137, engaging in negotiation that was functionally implicit as corrective feedback, but phonologically explicit in its encoding. This allowed SuJin to correct the error from line 136. She repeated the original targetlike option, and segmented the target-containing syllable to help isolate the form and increase its salience. Line 138 is an example of corrective feedback in which both the target form and negotiation move are implicitly encoded, as Park indicated continued noncomprehension. As the repetition he received in line 139 still was not convincing for him, in line 140 he juxtaposed both forms, implicitly asking for additional clarification, but through a move that was phonologically explicit. His interlocutor's response in line 141 is noteworthy in that she bypassed additional repetition of the form and opted for a metalinguistic description: "Simple," implying that she was saying the street name that they would both agree is easier to say, i.e. not including the difficult target form, /θ/. He accepted her explanation and they moved on.

Examples of both error types (speaker- and hearer-based) are visible in the following excerpt from Dyad 9:

258. Dong: (laughs) Uhl on da intersection, Sink, Sink Street?
259. Li-Xin: Think? ([sɪŋk]? *unclear*)
260. Dong: Yeah Sink. *Think.* Think Street?
261. Li-Xin: Wait a minute (3)
262. Dong: It's a east. (2)
263. Li-Xin: Ah. Thing:::
264. Dong: Yeah, Think.
265. Li-Xin: *Sink.*
266. Dong: Yeah.
267. Li-Xin: Or Think?
268. Dong: *Think* (2)
269. Li-Xin: Sink
270. Dong: Yeah.
271. Li-Xin: Ahah.
272. Dong: T-H. ([ti::eitš]) (*spelling the letters*)
273. Li-Xin: Ah! Think. Think.
[ ]
274. Dong: Hah.
275. Dong: Think. Think. Think
[ ]
276. Li-Xin: Think Street.
277. Dong: A::n Sree Town Avenue
278. Li-Xin: Three Town, okay.
279. Dong: Yeah.

Dong's modification from "sink" in line 258 to "think" in line 260 demonstrates realization of his own production error, after which he was very consistent with his articulation of /θ/. However, even once Dong's target form production had stabilized with greater targetlike accuracy, Li-Xin's ongoing corrective feedback, checking back and forth between the minimal pair options, shows an inability to identify what she was hearing, despite her apparent ability to orally produce both distinct forms. It was not until Dong resorts to spelling that Li-Xin finally indicated understanding, as she showed by her subsequent targetlike production in line 273. Ultimately, both participants provided and received corrective feedback, and provided modified output, the final result of which was targetlike perception and production of /θ/ for both as well. This corresponds well to Ellis' observation that "[i]n exchanges between learners, one learner's modified output is another learner's comprehensible input" (1999b, p. 14).

The vast majority of corrective feedback in this study was due to hearer-based errors, i.e. errors of perception, or at least uncertainty on the part of the hearer, not the speaker's lack of clarity in articulation. Most interlocutors demonstrated ability to produce the target form relatively consistently in the obligatory contexts of street names, but had greater difficulty with accurate perception. The task design itself may also have played a role in this, as there were two clearly available options, and either one had an equal chance of being correct at any given time. As there were no other contextual clues that would have helped the listener decipher the intended street name, it increased the listener's need to be absolutely certain about which option had been said. Thus, it is not surprising that, as the results in chapter 4 showed, most corrective feedback was phonologically explicit but implicitly negotiated, in the form of a confirmation check, as in line 259 above. This brings the discussion to the focus of research questions 1a and 2: corrective feedback.

CORRECTIVE FEEDBACK

Chapter 4 reported that nearly 75% of all corrective feedback contained an explicit phonological form and implicit negotiation move, mainly in the form of a confirmation check, which contained a repetition of either the target form or an alternative encoding. Confirmation checks, some of which are phonetically identical to a "repetition" (Lyster & Ranta, 1997) as forms of feedback, fall under this category, as outlined in chapter 2. As the map itself provides rather tight guidelines for discourse, as mentioned above, it is unsurprising that so few instances of corrective feedback contained explicit negotiation moves (23.8% total). As long as the form in question was included in the utterance (88.0% total), there remained little uncertainty regarding the cause of any breakdown in communication, at which point explicit negotiation moves may have been viewed as superfluous. Thus, learners typically chose to use the most verbally efficient means of signaling the breakdown.

Of the various types of explicit negotiation moves, task-based language occurred nearly twice as frequently (42.1%) as the second most widely-used strategy, which was in the form of direct requests. Again, this may be partially due to the nature of the task, as mentioned above. The prevalence of the direct request move (23.0%) is also notable, as it manifested as confirmation checks in the form of tag questions (e.g., "...right?"), and simple clarification requests (e.g., "say it again?"), both of which are very common discourse structures in native speakers' casual conversation. The topic of similarities between NS-NS and NNS-NNS discourse will be addressed later in this chapter.

In contrast to other corrective feedback types, metalinguistic feedback was surprisingly *un*common with only five tokens total: 2.8% of explicitly encoded negotiation moves, or 0.89% of the 559 total feedback moves identified. However, this was inevitably due, in part, to the methodology used to analyze the data of this study. As explained in chapter 3, this study separated metalanguage and overt negation as explicit *negotiation* move types, whereas other interaction studies combine them as a category of explicit *correction* (e.g.,

Lyster & Ranta, 1997), with metalanguage subsuming overt negation phrases like "no" and "not X" as pertaining to explicit corrective intent. If this study were to have combined them in this way as well, the metalinguistic total (including the 25 overt negation moves) would have been 16.8% of all the explicit negotiation moves. That would have made the metalinguistic strategy nearly equivalent in frequency to heralding (18.0%) in participants' interactions.

Although the frequencies of negotiation move types were not tallied for the minimal pair pre-task activity, it should be noted that all of these strategies were found – if to a lesser extent – in dyads' interaction on that activity as well. For example, after Hiroko and Peng of Dyad 17 got item #3 incorrect, Hiroko asked Peng to repeat both sentence options in line 30, "Can you say sentence-A?" She thereby demonstrated a feedback move that was phonologically explicit with explicit task-based language as well as a direct request. She then asked him to repeat sentence-B, in what appears to be a request for him to contrast the two forms for her. After a moment of confusion, the following exchange occurred (underlined words hereafter are only to assist the reader and hold no transcription-related function):

44.	Peng:	You mean I, I have to repeat sentence A?
45.	Hiroko:	A and B both.
46.	Peng:	Oh, okay. What a incredible oaf.
47.	Hiroko:	Mm.
48.	Peng:	What an incredible oath.
49.	Hiroko:	A::h...okay.
50.	Peng:	So, oath you can see th-th-th-th-th-th-th.
51.	Hiroko:	Mm.
52.	Peng:	And u::h...sound water in my mouth. You can hear it.
53.	Hiroko:	Okay.

Realizing his partner's difficulty hearing the difference, he granted her request and juxtaposed the two phrases for her to compare, then offered additional assistance. In line 50 he isolated the target phoneme multiple times, prefacing it with instructions including the target word and the attention-orienting phrase, "you can see." He then proceeded to provide metalinguistic input for her, describing the sound of the phoneme in line 52, which in his assessment includes a watery quality which he said she could hear. Thus, their exchange suggests that even decontextualized minimal pair activities such as this one can still have value as a catalyst for authentic, meaningful, and metalinguistically challenging communication between non-native speakers.

MODIFICATION

The task (and pre-task activity) not only facilitated attention to form by promoting corrective feedback, but the interactions revealed a plethora of opportunities for participants to modify their target form production with greater accuracy, which was the focus of research questions 1b and 3. It should be reiterated that only modifications that were related to street names were coded, though these were not the only points of miscommunication requiring negotiation. Although other modifications may have demonstrated attention to the target form, and may hold many other implications for SLA, the actual quantification of these episodes was beyond the scope of this study.

It was also important to distinguish when NNSs were truly attempting to modify their articulation of a single phoneme as opposed to accurately mirroring their partner's changes, as in Dyad 3's exchange below:

152. Ana: And when you find High <u>Path</u> Road?
153. Yumi:High *<u>Path</u>::?* Road. (1) Yes.
154. Ana: No, not High <u>Pat</u> Road, High <u>Pass</u> Road?
155. Yumi:Yeah. Ah High <u>Pass</u>? Road.
156. Ana: Yes?
157. Yumi:Mhm?

In this case, Ana, an L1-Spanish female, started telling Yumi, an L1-Japanese female, to go on High <u>Path</u> Road, which Yumi heard and carefully confirmed back to her, including higher intonation and gemination on the target form for increased salience. Ana then appeared to change her mind in line 154, with a nontargetlike (and likely L1-influenced) modification from [pæθ] to [pæt] for one street, and a deliberate juxtaposition and contrast to the newly selected minimal pair option, [pæs]. Yumi then heard and acknowledged the change and adjusted her own utterance accordingly. Thus, Yumi's contributions of corrective feedback were coded, but her change was not coded as an actual modification of form, as both of her utterances demonstrated accurate perception and production of each form that was presented to her. It is also worth noting that Ana was partially enabled to make the nontargetlike modification in line 154 because as long as the newly desired street name ("Pass") was pronounced clearly enough to be distinguishable from its alternative, the alternative ("Path") no longer needed to be targetlike, as long as the newly inaccurate articulation of /θ/ remained uniquely distinct from /s/. In other words, the essentialness of the target form's accuracy had been lost, thereby allowing her to attend to other aspects of the exchange without sacrificing successful communication.

A second issue to address is that the tallying of targetlike and nontargetlike modifications did not take into account the difference between what will be referred to as “backsliding,” vs. “blind” nontargetlike (-) modification. Backsliding, in this study, refers to a temporary reversion to (-) articulation after a previous (+) modification of the same word, *not* a modification toward the interlocutor’s own nontargetlike *theta* production that differed from the speaker’s nontargetlike articulation. Although there were indeed many modifications that started from a targetlike form and changed to a less targetlike form, it must be realized that many times it was the same dyad revisiting the same street and readdressing the same struggles, as an early (+) modification may have shown temporary attention to form, but not complete automatization. It is thus not surprising that additional rounds of negotiation regarding the same street name were necessary, as once again speakers reverted to habitual, nontargetlike production (-) after having reached greater accuracy previously, and then needed to renegotiate to reach targetlike production again. The (+)/(-) patterns may be a potential indicator of awareness of the NNS’s lack of control of a form and efforts to increase that control.

“Blind” (-) modification, in contrast, often occurred in more random patterns that seemed to indicate that the speaker not only did not realize when he had made a (-) modification (as backsliding was also a subconscious modification), but also was unaware when he had made a (+) modification, i.e. the NNS not only lacked control of the target form, but was unaware of his own articulatory changes in *either* direction.

An example of backsliding is visible in the following excerpt from Dyad 9:

197. Li-Xin:	Ahah. Okay, Sor, s, serv, serv, way an <u>North, Norse</u> Man's
198. Dong:	Yeah
199. Li-Xin:	Alley.
200. Dong:	Yeah.
201. Li-Xin:	Okay (2) Uh, you can keep, keep going to the south?
202. Dong:	Yeah?
203. Li-Xin:	On <u>North, Norse</u> Man Alley.

Li-Xin’s habitual /s/ production was originally more dentalized and less strident than standard, closer to a variant of [θ], but her /θ/ position was not interdental enough to be sufficiently targetlike either, resulting in a sound that was virtually identical to her version of /s/. Through the negotiations, she worked to distinguish both phonemes in their respective ways. As the starting point had previously been established as Norse Man's Alley (verified), line 197 shows a habitual (-) change to "North" (which also may be influenced by hyper-sensitized overgeneralization due to the task design) and immediate (+) to "Norse" upon hearing and recognizing her own error. The same pattern occurs in line 203.

After having been corrected by her partner several times in earlier stages of the task, Li-Xin was now self-correcting and making her /s/ more strident, so the changes *to* a variant of "North" are (-) and represent backsliding to her default nontargetlike production, whereas her changes to "Norse" (+) are her own recognition of her error and efforts at immediate self modification, showing greater effort and success at targetlike control of the form.

While it appears that the number of (-) and (+) modifications cancel each other out in averages in this excerpt, findings in chapter 4 showed that there were nearly twice as many (+) modifications as (-). Ultimately, it is argued that these findings overall, exemplified by this exchange, is indeed indicative of phonological *resensitization,* i.e. retraining the neurosensory perception and production mechanisms to detect and distinguish between new phonological contrasts to which they had otherwise been 'de-tuned' after years or decades of L1-limited routines. As mentioned in chapter 1, resensitization is an essential step in adult L2 pronunciation learning; thus, this evidence of resensitization challenges the absoluteness of the relationship between fossilization and the notion of "critical periods" in L2 phonology.

Self-initiated Modification

As mentioned in chapter 2, self-initiated, or non-pushed modification can be just as valuable for SLA as pushed modification, as is visible in the previous example. In this task, self-initiated modifications were surprisingly common, and nearly always resulted in something more targetlike, i.e. demonstrating greater control, than the original utterance. Sometimes, it may simply be that the speaker heard or felt a mistake in her own utterance via auditory or proprioceptive feedback as soon as it was said, and recognized the need to correct it. This may have been the case in the previous example. Alternatively, self-initiated modification may manifest itself as a form of hypothesis testing, as demonstrated several times in the excerpt that opened this chapter. Hypothesis testing, as a component of output processing (Swain, 1998) also has the side benefit of making a language form more salient via repetition or contrast, as in the following excerpt from Yan-Fu in an utterance from a longer exchange, as shown below:

210. Yan-Fu: to the… Theme, mm, Thene, Theme, eh, Theme Park Drive.

Although the final nasal consonant in "Theme" seemed to be at least part of the challenge the speaker was trying to resolve, it allowed the listener four chances to hear the target form and identify it as different from its minimal pair street name, "Team Park Drive," thereby reducing the need for additional corrective feedback.

Similarly, although quantification and analysis of utterances such as "go souse... I mean thouth, uh, south" were beyond the scope of this study, as mentioned above, they are clearly instances of attention to the target form, and hold valuable implications for the field of SLA. They may actually provide even greater evidence of steps toward automatization than the negotiations surrounding street names: they demonstrate awareness of the need for the target form in obligatory contexts and progress toward increasing control thereof *despite* the lack of a minimal pair word or other condition that would require accurate production as essential for successful task completion.

This evidence lends additional credence to the value of dyadic interaction in L2 pronunciation acquisition, regardless of the L1 of the interlocutors, and may even support the notion that non-native speakers would be more likely to draw each other's attention to some target forms than a NS interlocutor would be. This is because, as also addressed in chapter 2, NNSs tend to negotiate more when working with each other, whereas a NS might be more likely to simply provide the correction, and thus not require the NNS to work to increase the intelligibility of his utterance; alternatively, the NNS may be more likely to simply defer to the NS and not want to outwardly admit or address each instance of noncomprehension.

Evidence of Increased Control in Listening Comprehension

"Targetlike modification" has been operationalized in this study as demonstrating steps toward acquisition of *control* of a form, including using it when it is necessary as well as avoiding it when it is NOT necessary. However, in addition to helping students attain more targetlike production, there was also abundant evidence of learners honing their listening skill accuracy, as they focused on their articulation. When the NNSs could not understand each other despite articulatory accuracy, they used repetition, rephrasing, and other strategies (discussed below) in their negotiations around the target form in this task. As they did so, they appeared to provide each other with abundant input for processing and numerous opportunities to expand their aural skills, helping each other aurally distinguish the target form from its commonly substituted alternatives and pushing each other to select and articulate the obligatory form in a given context.

Chapter 1 addressed several issues regarding the relationship between perception and production in L2 phonology, but "modification of perception," per se, is sometimes more difficult to operationalize and code. As the data revealed, sometimes the participants would think aloud, at which point it was easier to see when they were noticing a difference. However, sometimes the only way to verify that the listener had gone from misunderstanding to understanding was by context, such as having landed on the right intersection number for the final destination on the map, which demonstrated that they did understand a previously negotiated street name. This is revealed in the following exchange from Mehmet and Yu-Shan in Dyad 13:

212. Mehmet:	Up to::::::... Thee, Theme Park Drive.
213. Yu-Shan:	Theme Park Drive?
214. Mehmet:	Mm.
215. Yu-Shan:	Team or Theme?
216. Mehmet:	T, uh Theme, yes.
217. Yu-Shan:	Okay.
218. Mehmet:	Just uh on:::
219. Yu-Shan:	On the::: corner?
220. Mehmet:	Left you, yes the corner.
221. Yu-Shan:	Oh, the forty-three.
222. Mehmet:	Yeah!

In this case, Yu-Shan, the hearer, gives corrective feedback in lines 213 and 215. Mehmet repeats the keyword, "Theme," but Yu-Shan's last response is simply "Okay" in line 217. She never explicitly confirms the word herself after juxtaposing the two forms as part of her feedback move. As a result, it is not immediately clear if she truly understood until line 221, when she finally says she is at intersection #43 (the intersection of Theme Park Drive and Coral Wreath Lane.) Thus, her response in line 221 suggests that she has gone from uncertainty (lines 213 & 215) to comprehension, or that her perception has changed. That Yu-Shan had been able to articulate both forms clearly, was seen in both instances of corrective feedback. Thus, this negotiation routine suggests that the task can impact auditory processes such as perception and discrimination in addition to focusing on pronunciation and oral production, all of which are essential processes in L2 phonological development, and in SLA overall.

Additional Strategies and the Role of Task-Based Interaction

In addition to corrective feedback and modification in general, this study identified several other strategies that learners used to draw each other's attention to phonological target forms. Some of these were related to communication and interaction at the level of message transmission, while others were directly related to the tasks in which the NNSs engaged. For example, the vocally-oriented strategies found in table 4.3, specifically gemination, pausing, intonation and volume contrasts, segmentation and schwa-epenthesis, represent a type of interactional modification. They do not modify the articulatory features of the target (or contrast) form itself, but rather manipulate its relationship to other forms in the immediate phonetic environment in ways that will increase its salience. Minimal pair juxtaposition helps to isolate the target and contrast forms, and their syntactic proximity to each other makes the contrast more salient.

These strategies are of interest for various reasons. First, they were frequently combined with each other, e.g. juxtaposition with gemination, or – most commonly – pausing with intonation changes. Second, they occurred both in corrective feedback moves as well as in modifications, and thus perhaps their role should not be erroneously limited as a subcategory of corrective feedback alone. Third, they often occurred preemptively, in non-pushed clarification efforts in *anticipation* and *avoidance* of possible miscommunication, once participants recognized the linguistic target of the task. Long categorized this type of move as a "strategic negotiation device," in contrast to "tactical negotiation devices" which are used to repair miscommunication that has already occurred (1996, p. 418, p. 418). As the strategies from table 4.3 were employed to enhance the functions of both "strategic" and "tactical" negotiation devices, perhaps they can more generally be classified as "highlighting moves." However, due to the inherent design of the map task, the distinction between what is proactive/"strategic"[18] and reactive/"tactical" is blurred.

Once participants realize the task-essentialness of the target form, *theta*, it could be argued that all "highlighting" of utterances that include the target form are reactive in nature. Rather than reacting to their interlocutor's speech, even "strategic"/proactively modified utterances are essentially participants' reactions to the linguistic demands of the task. They are acknowledging the need for accuracy in oral and aural distinction between the phonemic contrasts in context, and are thus trying to help their partners avoid the pitfalls of potential miscommunication that await them literally at every turn. "Strategic" pre/post-target pausing, raised volume or intonation, gemination, etc. were often used when giving directions from the very first time the name of a street was uttered, without first having been pushed for any clarification. Thus, the design of the task is once again seen to influence participants' linguistic behavior.

Overgeneralization, Obligatory Context and Task Essentialness

For many participants, their attention had not only been oriented to the target form through this task, but they also found themselves overgeneralizing the inclusion of *theta* in otherwise non-obligatory contexts, combining it with one of the alternative forms, or transposing it with other phonemes. This error occurred in various contexts, such as directional/orientation phrases:

---

18 "Strategic" moves, in quotation marks, will specifically connote Long's interpretation as contrasted with "tactical" moves. Otherwise, any references to strategic moves in general will connote a more general interpretation of the word, as used throughout the rest of this study, such as with references to strategic schwa-epenthesis.

Dyad 5, line 18
Byoung-Gon: [...] you can go the thous ([θaus]) [...]

Dyad 7, line 134
Tsin-Hua: Walk thouth ([θauθ]) until, Faithful Way.

Dyad 7, line 176
Hae-Ryu: You just keep go:::... just go::: sthouth ([sθauθ]).

Dyad 3, line 137
Yumi: Yes. So, number twenty-theven?

Such overextension also occurred in street names, but in positions that did not pertain to a minimal pair, e.g.:

Dyad 5, line 229
Byoung-Gon: M:::, you can go, sous. Until, Thfathful:: ([θfæθful::])... Faithful Way.

Dyad 8, line 190
JunHee: [...] an, um, nor Nors::e, Manth, ah! No. Norse Man's Alley.

Dyad 12, Line 281
JaeWon: [...] Until, Norse? Manth Alley. North, Northə Man's Alley.

It should be noted that the speakers here had not otherwise shown evidence of any type of lisp, with the possible exception of HaeRyu from Dyad 7. But in her nontargetlike utterance above, [sθauθ], her effort at distinguishing /s/ and /θ/ is visible, manifesting itself as two sequential phonemes, possibly showing an initial attempt to exert greater control over the lisp and produce a more strident /s/ but relaxing that control before moving to the subsequent vowel.

More importantly, in the examples pertaining to street names, despite the lack of minimal pair confusion due to the location of the overgeneralization, speakers still realized their own errors and immediately self-corrected with greater accuracy and control of use. Specifically, this strategy included omitting the /θ/ in otherwise nonobligatory contexts in all three examples above. The first showed recognition that it *was* needed, as well as in which position: specifically, prior to the word-medial /f/, but not the word-initial /f/. The final example shows the speaker having originally included it in the coda of the wrong word, switching both codas to make them more targetlike, and even strategically epenthesizing a schwa after the obligatory *theta* to help increase the salience of the correction.

A recurring pattern among the seven examples above is that in the examples in which targetlike accuracy was not essential to successful task completion, the overgeneralization was not modified. In fact, most participants were very careful regarding accuracy when pronouncing street names, which provides much evidence in support of the need for a tightly designed task-target relationship (Loschky & Bley-Vroman, 1993; Pica et al., 1993). However, despite the overwhelming presence of *theta* and need for its accuracy in some contexts, often *theta* was not pronounced in a targetlike way in other words that contained *theta* but without minimal pair alternatives, as in the following example from Yu-Shan and Mehmet in Dyad 13:

88. Yu-Shan:	Boot Road and Coral, Wreath Lane, intersection.
89. Mehmet:	Okay now, so you go north, un, you go north until Third Way. Thro, Theorem Way.
90. Yu-Shan:	Therom.
91. Mehmet:	Yeah, Theorom Way.
93. Yu-Shan:	Theorom Way.
(11 turns)	
105. Mehmet:	[...] Can you guess a number?
106. Yu-Shan:	Sree? ([sri:])
107. Mehmet:	Yes, it's three.
108. Yu-Shan:	Okay, sree. ([sri:])

This type of occurrence shows that no matter how well a task orients NNSs' attention to a target form, the likelihood of learners noticing the form may be greatly reduced when not linked directly to meaning. As such, these examples also demonstrate the limits of attentional "orientation," and thereby support its subordination to "detection" as a level of attention necessary for noticing (Tomlin & Villa, 1994). The task was designed to orient participants' attention to the target form, i.e. to precondition their receptivity toward it, as defined in chapter 1. Yet despite such efforts at attentional preconditioning and alignment, even after having negotiated multiple *theta*-inclusive street names, participants often – though not always – reverted to focusing on meaning rather than form in contexts in which target form essentialness was not required for successful task completion.

Orthographic Influence

The influence of orthography was also visible in the NNSs' task performance. As predicted in chapter 3, Coral Wreath Lane was the most problematic. Part of the cause may have been lack of familiarity with the word "wreath" and even the object it semantically represents, at which point participants were not looking at the word as a singular concept, but rather as nothing more than a series of sounds to be strung together. This may be related to Gorsuch's claims about the influence of unknown vocabulary and customs on test validity (2001), as mentioned in chapter 3. Despite the fact that the researcher modeled all street names after passing out the map, allowing everyone to repeat and practice the names, ask for help on any particularly difficult ones, and take notes to help them remember, there was still a variety of nontargetlike versions of "wreath" that distinguished it from the alternative street's name, "Coral Reef Lane." These variations included [wreas], where all "silent" letters were assigned sound; [wes], eliding the 'r' completely and voicing the 'w' instead; and [wels] or (less frequently) [welθ], perhaps confusing "wreath" with the word "wealth" which may appear phonetically and orthographically similar, particularly with the 'L/R' confusion many Asian students encounter. Unfortunately, almost all of these variations allowed participants to clearly convey their street intention to their interlocutor without requiring targetlike articulation of /θ/.

Theme Park Drive also caused some unexpected problems, in two ways. First, several participants referred to it as "Seem" [sim] or "Seemy" [simi] Park Drive, not only with L1-influenced substitution of [s] for /θ/, but by vocalizing the word-final 'silent-e.' Conversely, some participants made reference to [tema] Park Drive. This occasionally caused confusion, as it could have referred to either Theme Park Drive or Team Park Drive. First, that combination of phonemes, though out of order, would appear to represent the spelling of the word "Team."

This transposition of phonemes may also reflect L1 influence, but because the translation of the word "theme," shared by many languages, is commonly pronounced [tema], which is a Latin cognate in Spanish, and a borrowed word in Korean and Japanese, for example.

However, there is additional evidence of resensitization/re-tuning of their sound-symbol associations, as mentioned in chapter 1, in participants' metacognitive comments. For example, JunHee and SoYoung in Dyad 8 had a problem with Theme Park Drive, which resolved itself as follows:

82.	JunHee:	Oh yeah. Okay? (2) ha, pa (*singing*). I wanna go Reeding Terminal?
83.	SoYoung:	Yes?
84.	JunHee:	From:::, Steel Symbol Court, and, Tem, De, Tem, Temeh? Tema Park Drive? (1)
85.	SoYoung:	Uh, you mean Steel Symbol Court and [Tem, *Theme*] Park Drive, right?
86.	JunHee:	[Tema? Thim? Tim?]
87.	JunHee:	Uh, Symbol

88. SoYoung: Steel Symbol Court and Theme park drive right?
89. JunHee: Theme yeah not team. [xxx]
[ ]
90. SoYoung: Yes. Um::: (2) Yes, so::::.
91. SoYoung: You can
92. JunHee: Theme, theme, ah, forgot again okay (← *talking quietly to herself*)

In this case, JunHee's think-aloud in line 92 demonstrates a heightened awareness of her own errors for which she admonished herself. This may be evidence that such focused task participation can also help to improve learners' understanding of the relationship between orthography and pronunciation.

Similarly, Dyad 5 encountered a communication breakdown as early as line 48, in which Byoung-Gon (L1-Korean male) directed his partner to Ticket lane, repeating the street name several times, to which his partner, Sachiko (L1-Japanese female), simply replied "Yeah," but ultimately guessed corner #50 (Thicket Lane and Truce Alley), which shows she had misunderstood. They started over and 48 turns later (line 96) he again said, "Ticket Lane," and this time she repeated, "Ticket Lane, yeah" (line 97), as shown below. They agreed on the pronunciation, (confirmed by the researcher and second coder as well), not realizing that they were looking at different streets until line 99 when she guessed intersection #49, (Thicket Lane and Truth Alley). It was not until line 102 that they started to get to the bottom of the issue:

96. Byoung-Gon: Anda, you can make a right? T, Ticket… Ticket Lane.
97. Sachiko: Ticket Lane, yeah.
98. Byoung-Gon: Yeah. (2)
99. Sachiko: Forty-nine? (2) (laughs)
100. Byoung-Gon: No.
101. Sachiko: You said Tru:::-
102. Byoung-Gon: Tic, not, not, not, not, Th::::ick. Ticket, Ticket.
103. Sachiko: Ticket.
104. Byoung-Gon: Not Thicket.
105. Sachiko: A:::h!
106. Byoung-Gon: Ticket Lane.
107. Sachiko: Okay okay okay okay. I misunderstood. Ticket.
108. Byoung-Gon: Yeah Ticket just Ticket.
109. Sachiko: So:::, is it, uh::, fifty-eight?
110. Byoung-Gon: Okay.

The orthography/phonology confusion may have occurred as a result of the specific pair of words. Although Japanese speakers typically substitute [s] for /θ/ rather than [t], they also typically associate the orthographic syllable "ti" with the affricate [tši] when learning to write Japanese words in Romanized script (*romaji,*) usually before learning English, as Japanese only has /tši/, not /ti/, as part of the moraic inventory. Thus, having potentially assigned frication to "Ticket" through subconscious L1-influence, Sachiko may have accepted the non-fricative [ti] as accurate by default for "Thicket."

Regardless of the exact nature or cause of these miscommunications, many if not most of the problems negotiated were resolved with interlocutors reaching consensus on a more targetlike pronunciation of whichever street they had chosen, thereby overcoming the orthographic obstacles, and learning to associate more accurate articulation patterns with the spelling patterns they observed.

MORE THAN JUST "UNAWARE"

In a few instances it became clear that one of the interlocutors truly could not hear the difference between *theta* and another form; they not only seemed to lack any awareness that what they were producing and what they *thought* they were producing were not identical, but seemed adamant that any confusion was their interlocutor's fault. A greater challenge arises when one person thinks she's saying one thing but (per everyone else's indications, NS and NNS alike) it seems like she is articulating something else. In pair 20, for example, Hung-Yi (L1-Chinese female) attempts to lead Ikue (L1-Japanese female) to intersection 59, on Mossy Hill Street, at which point the following exchange occurs, beginning with Ikue's confirmation check:

114.	Ikue:	Mossy, Mossy Hill Street?
115.	Hung-Yi:	eh, Moss-
116.	Ikue:	Mossy
117.	Hung-Yi:	not Mossy! Mossy, Mossy Hill Street, M-
118.	Ikue:	Moth-Mothy Hill Street it first one
119.	Hung-Yi:	yeah
120.	Ikue:	uh, fifty, fifty-first
121.	Hung-Yi:	yeah, Mossy not Frothy!

Hung-Yi misperceives Ikue's targetlike /s/ use, and attempts to correct her quite explicitly in line 117 using what appears to be an attempt at juxtaposition, except that there is no discernable phonetic difference between the attempts she makes. This confuses her interlocutor and causes more subsequent problems than it resolves. Shortly thereafter, they realize they are still in the wrong location and the negotiation continues.

In such a situation, there is still room for gain, as a NNS with the aforementioned limitations will force his or her interlocutor to use additional strategies for success in message clarification. From a research perspective, these strategies will be visible, as in lines 114, 116 and 118 above. Additionally, learners with such limitations in perception or production will still be able to use various strategies to draw their interlocutors' attention to form, as in lines 117 and 121 above.

When the problem is due to something more related to speech pathology than SLA, such as a lisp, the problem is compounded, as it may go beyond aforementioned L1-influenced de-tuning. For example, in Dyad 7, Tsin-Hua, an L1-Chinese female, appeared to give her partner, HaeRyu, an L1-Korean female, directions to Truth (not Truce) Alley. She even provided a segmentation of not only the target-form-containing syllable, but isolated the individual segment multiple times in line 265 (bold type indicates loud voices):

261. Tsin-Hua:	I'm in da:::... uh:::... inter::section? of... chu, chru::ce? Alley. *(/θ/?/s/? unclear)*
262. HaeRyu:	Truce?
263. Tsin-Hua:	Truth.
264. HaeRyu:	Could you tell me again?
265. Tsin-Hua:	Truth? Th, th, th, (*laughs*)
266. HaeRyu:	(*laughs*)
267. Tsin-Hua:	***Truth*** Alley.
268. HaeRyu:	***Truthə***?
269. Tsin-Hua:	No, ***Truth***. *(Thinks she's saying Truce? Non-strident quality to final phoneme; sounds like /θ/.)*
270. HaeRyu:	Truce?
271. Tsin-Hua:	Yeah.
272. HaeRyu:	Okay.

In such a case, Tsin-Hua's modification went from something neither /θ/ nor /s/ toward a much clearer *theta,* despite apparently wanting to articulate the alternative, /s/. HaeRyu's changes, however, were not actually changes to a given phoneme, but switching from one option to the other, as clarification requests/confirmation checks on perception to see which her partner was actually trying to say. In the end, HaeRyu needed to give "multiple choice" options, at which point she could be more certain that she was producing the two distinct words in the minimal pair, and allowed her interlocutor to select the one that matched her own (Tsin-Hua's) intention, which, in the end, appeared to be "Truce Alley."[19]

19 This excerpt was played for an audience of six NS PhD candidates and a NS professor. All unanimously believed Tsin-Hua was saying "Truth," as became evident at the end upon

In the end, whether the problem is rooted in SLA or speech pathology, for any significant targetlike acquisition to take place, a person demonstrating such challenges would probably need individual instruction with a teacher or speech pathologist to recognize her nontargetlike speech patterns in contrast to what targetlike speech would entail. In particular, if it were deemed to be a problem more akin to speech pathology – whether the person were a NS or NNS, at that point – multi-media and/or multi-sensory information pertaining to the contrast would probably be necessary for any true awareness of targetlike vs. nontargetlike production and perception. Some tools could include mirrors, recording their own voices in order to hear themselves objectively for analysis, and computer generated visual displays of their own vocal recordings, such as on a spectrograph. Realistically, all learners can benefit from these interventions (de Bot, 1980), but they will be even more essential when working with learners with speech impediments, or who otherwise seem less able to recognize their own patterns at all through more traditional instructional approaches.

SOUNDING LIKE EACH OTHER

Research questions aside, the question for which more people will likely want to have an answer is whether or not participants ultimately picked up each other's nontargetlike habits and "ended up sounding like each other." It is encouraging to be able to state that, according to the data, this was almost never the case. In actuality, participants rarely assimilated each other's unique non-targetlike productions of the target form. On the occasion such nontargetlike pronunciation was appropriated, it was generally done to facilitate task completion by *temporarily borrowing* the interlocutor's phonetic production pattern if the hearer seemed unable to otherwise distinguish the minimal pairs when more targetlike options were produced.

For example in Dyad 26, the street Theme Park Drive caused initial difficulty, but over the course of the entire task, the problem was resolved for both participants. Temporarily, Bai-Ling (L1-Chinese female) started out with targetlike articulation of "Theme" ([θim]), but chose to modify it in a nontargetlike way (-) to match more closely to Akiko's (L1-Japanese female) first nontargetlike articulation in line 114, [šim]:

113. Bai-Ling: [...] Steel Symbol Court and Theme Park Drive.
114. Akiko: Sheme Park Drive ok?
115. Bai-Ling: Seem Park Drive.

---

hearing lines 270-271 which identified the actual street as "Truce Alley," at which point everyone present let out shocked responses of "Oh!' or "What?!" in unison.

A few moments later the street was revisited, and this time orthography appeared to play a greater role, as Bai-Ling seemed to vocalize the 'silent-e' at the end of "Theme":

133. Bai-Ling: until uh... seem, Seemy, Seemy Park Dry. Seemy Park Dry.
134. Akiko: ok
135. Bai-Ling: Seemy Seemy Park Dry.
136. Akiko: ok

Approximately 100 turns later the street was again revisited. This time in line 238 Bai-Ling demonstrated modified, targetlike production (+) of "Theme" but then immediately reverted to the form that, perhaps, she thought her partner would more easily understand:

238. Bai-Ling: […] and uh, uh Theme?, and uh and uh… Seemy Park Drive.
239. Akiko: Seemy Park Drive.
240. Bai-Ling: Seem, Park Drive (5) Mossy.
241. Akiko: Mothy?
242. Bai-Ling: Mossy
243. Akiko: Mossy, and…

Bai-Ling quickly re-modified to a more targetlike articulation of the word by dropping the word-final epenthetic /i/, and although there seemed to be some question and vacillation on both interlocutors' parts over the course of the next ten turns, they both ultimately resolved the discussion with targetlike perception and production of the form in question:

244. Bai-Ling: Mossy Hill Stree, and… and uh Theme? th, Theme? Park Drive.
245. Akiko: Seem Park Drive… ok
246. Bai-Ling: Mossy
247. Akiko: Mossy
248. Bai-Ling: Mossy, Mossy Hill Mossy Hill Street and uh Seem Park Drive.
249. Akiko: Theme Seem Theme?
250. Bai-Ling: Seem Theme
251. Akiko: Theme.
252. Bai-Ling: Theme Park Dry.
253. Akiko: Ok… […]

Finally, 180 turns later on the very last route, Akiko chose Theme Park Drive and High Path Road as her starting point, which Bai-Ling needed to confirm:

433.	Bai-Ling:	And uh <u>Team</u> Park Drive?
434.	Akiko:	Yes
435.	Bai-Ling:	High *Pass* ro
436.	Akiko:	<u>*Theme*</u> Park dribe. Theme? Park dribe.
437.	Bai-Ling:	<u>Theme</u> Park Drive and uh High *Path*::: ro?
438.	Akiko:	yes
439.	Bai-Ling:	<u>Theme</u> Park Drive and uh High Path ro, you can go east

This time, although she first produced "Team Park Drive," her quick switch to Theme Park Drive (with intonation change for emphasis as part of a clarification request) was immediately targetlike. As such, for this route, both interlocutors' production of "Theme" was targetlike, and neither seemed to feel the need to substitute [sim] or [simi].

Thus, despite temporary mutual distraction from targetlike articulation in the beginning of the task, both interlocutors were able to push each other in a step towards automatization of the target form, *theta*. The argument could be made that negotiation and modification might lessen by the end of a task because participants have simply grown accustomed to each other's speech patterns, whether targetlike, similar to their own, or completely distinct. However, the above example demonstrates that not only is it untrue that learners will inevitably learn each other's mistakes, but that they can indeed push each other toward more targetlike production and perception, helping each other resensitize/re-tune their sensitivities to new phonemic contrasts.

The Task, Revisited

A Task by Any Other Name...

But was the map task, in effect, a "task" (Pica et al., 1993) or merely an exercise in minimal pair distinction? Analysis of transcripts consistently showed evidence of it being a true communication task, in which participants had identified a common goal, and were working together by requesting and providing information to each other in order to reach that goal. As mentioned in the introduction to the section on modification, learners negotiated many different items through the course of their interaction, not only those which pertained to the target form.

A somewhat entertaining example of this phenomenon occurred with Dyad 2, in which Alicia, whose L1 was Spanish, was trying to direct her partner, Ul-Sik (L1-Korean male) to Boot Road, but pronounced it, "Wot" Road. (Presumably due to L1 influence, the evolution from the phonological /bu:t/ to the phonetic product [wot] may have followed a sequence akin to: /bu:t/ → /bot/ (orthographic influence) → /ßot/ → /wot/.) Unfortunately for her interlocutor, "Wot Road" sounds essentially the same as "what road," and the resulting exchange almost literally followed Abbott and Costello's classic "Who's on First" comedy routine[20] (specifically relating to the fictitious second baseman, whose name was supposedly "What,"):

16. Alicia: In High Pat Road you need turn right? Of est? To Wot Road?
[ ]
17. Ul-Sik: Yeah
18. Ul-Sik: To what road?
19. Alicia: Wot Road.
20. Ul-Sik: U::h
21. Alicia: Do you see dis. You need… Ah, Wot Road, de first is Woth, Road? And de nes is Boat? Road.
22. Ul-Sik: M:::, u::h…

She did accurately modify her word-initial /b/ by the end of the routine, referring to the target street as [bot] Road instead of [wot] Road, though the minimal pair street "Booth Road" was also pronounced with a word-initial [w], [woθ] Road. The irony is that the target form, /θ/, and its minimal pair alternative, /t/, were the *only* phonemes produced *accurately* in the street names in question right from the start.

Influences of the Task Itself

Having established the validity of the map task, a few of the influences of its design on participant interaction should be addressed. Several have been mentioned already throughout this chapter. To summarize: first, the existence of minimal pairs may have increased the proportion of hearer-based negotiations since there were two viable options the speaker could have chosen at all times. Second, the task successfully balanced communicative requirement and task-essentialness of form in order to ensure maximum negotiation of form and meaning; however, keeping discourse naturalistic while controlling its range to increase form-essentialness (Loschky & Bley-Vroman, 1993) most likely influenced the heavy proportion of corrective feedback moves in which the negotiation intent was implicit, though the phonological form in question was explicit (i.e. moves that were classified as PE-NI). Third, in *reaction* to the task design, participants used many *proactive* ("strategic") highlighting moves once they understood the linguistic target embedded in the task and the challenges posed by the minimal pair names.

20 This comparison is dedicated to my father.

In addition, the task was found to provide a type of corrective feedback to the dyad, identifying miscommunication that neither interlocutor had recognized. In particular, at the end of a "route," if the person following directions landed on the wrong intersection number, it then became obvious that there had been miscommunication on one of the two intersecting street names, and additional negotiation was required. This finding also is in line with Pica, Kanagy and Falodun's (1993) assertion that one of the task criteria most likely to ensure maximal negotiation was if there was only one possible correct answer on which the interlocutors had to agree.

The controlled discourse of the task design also succeeded in providing an important context to holding the target form essential to successful task completion. When the target form was found in word- or syllable-final position, some participants' propensity for coda-deletion created an ambiguity of meaning, as "High [pa] Road" could just as easily have referred to High *Path* Road or High *Pass* Road, if there was no other context from which the listener could recover the intended form. While such issues of recoverability (Weinberger, 1987) originally were found to explain intralearner variation on more- and less- formal language "tasks," as mentioned in chapter 1, the map task used in this study succeeded in retaining and utilizing this condition discouraging ambiguity, but in an otherwise communicative, "informal" context.

One final design-related issue that occasionally "thwarted" maximal negotiation opportunity could be seen when students forgot or deliberately violated some of the rules of the task, such as the "no numbers must be used when giving directions" rule. Dyad 3, for example, repeatedly incorporated phrases such as, "On the first street you find..." Thus, the listener could occasionally have ignored the street name completely and still arrived at the target destination. Fortunately, outside of Dyad 3, this was a very infrequent occurrence, and typically was used as a last resort. However, it clearly demonstrated the essentialness of establishing the right task conditions in order for the linguistic and interactional objectives of the task to be realized.

LIMITATIONS AND DIRECTIONS FOR FUTURE RESEARCH

With any study, there are limitations to its methodology and scope of application, but ideally these limitations will open doors to avenues of further inquiry. In the map task used in this study, a possible influence on the number of verifiable theta-inclusive streets selected for destination points as well as routes may have been the order of the streets on the map. The intended map design tried to (a) mix minimal pair sets using /s/, /t/ and /f/; (b) mix minimal pairs with the target form in word initial-, medial- and final position as much as possible; and (c) alternate whether the theta-inclusive name or alternative name was listed first. However, it is possible that a different order of streets could have yielded a different proportion of theta-inclusive streets traversed, and thus inspired a different number of negotiation moves and modifications.

Regarding participants, surprisingly, a noteworthy number of participants in this study demonstrated some form of frontal lisp, whether mild, with a slightly less strident /s/, or profound, in which the /s/ manifested as a full *theta* ([θ]) each time. This may be due to many causes, such as an underbite or crooked teeth alignment, particularly along the top teeth allowing breath to escape more freely whereby reducing the strident feature of [s], resulting in a phonetic product more like the *theta*. As the vast majority of the participants were from countries where cosmetic dentistry—e.g., using braces to straighten children's teeth for 'picture-perfect' smiles—is far less common than here in the US, this hypothesis is not unreasonable.[21] Regardless of the cause, the high proportion of participants with a nonstandard, nonstrident or dentalized [s] production undoubtedly had an impact on the data, specifically in the nature and number of negotiations and modifications needed to make /θ/ vs. /s/ control more targetlike.

More importantly, as this study was a process-oriented study, there was no attempt to measure acquisition. However, as it became clear through the analysis of the interactions in this study, NNSs can indeed draw each other's attention to form via corrective feedback and other verbal strategies, as well as push each other toward greater accuracy and control of targeted phonemes. Thus, in the future, a pre-test and post-test assessment of participants' accuracy of perception and production of the target form before and after participating on this map task could provide additional support for its value as a pedagogic and research tool.

An additional methodological issue concerns the lack of linguistic analysis tools such as computer generated spectrographs to more mathematically measure phonetic modification. As this study was primarily about NNS-NNS interaction, what was most important was whether such modifications were targetlike enough to be discernable to an interlocutor. But how much modification is "enough"? Presumably, if it were discernable to a NNS interlocutor, it would also be discernable to a NS transcriber/coder, at which point it would be considered *sufficiently* more/less targetlike to be quantified. Realistically, the "gray" area of modifications that were indeed effected but not enough so as to

21 Dental conditions have been found to influence other studies as well. "The relatively poor teeth of Japanese people played a curious role in the X-ray microbeam project. When the first one was built in Tokyo," (in the 1960s and 70s), "it was unable to distinguish between the radio-opaque pellets used as targets and fillings. (The higher-powered one in Wisconsin was built in part to overcome this problem.) Because it was so hard to find Japanese people with no fillings, in spite of the location of the machine in Tokyo, most of the data collected was for English." (B. Poser, personal communication, January 21, 2008). Such dental issues, particularly of older generations, were confirmed by O. Fujimura, who conducted phonological research as part of the original microbeam project in Tokyo (personal correspondence, January 22, 2008).

be noticeable to "the naked ear," per se, may include modifications that were neither more (+) nor less (-) targetlike, but merely nontargetlike in other ways. The data would inevitably raise the number of types and tokens of modifications recorded, and provide excellent fodder for deeper, more comprehensive analysis of the range of what learners are capable of doing when participating on such tasks, but such analysis was ultimately beyond the scope of this study.

A final issue pertains to the lack of a NS baseline. An observation was made by several colleagues during the data analysis phase of this study: part of what makes the additionally identified strategies (e.g. intonation and juxtaposition) interesting is that they are probably more like typical discourse strategies between native speakers when giving directions or other potentially confusing information. For example, in giving directions, it would not be uncommon to have the following conversation:

A: Take Walnut Street west to Fifteenth Street.
B: Fif*teenth,* Street or *Fif*tieth Street?
A: Fif*teenth.*

Native speakers of English inherently use a higher pitch/intonation or volume contrast to emphasize the item in question, pause after it to raise its salience and provide processing time for the listener, and juxtapose the alternatives when the confusion is due to a binary choice. Similarly, when ordering merchandise over the telephone, a commonly experienced exchange has been along the lines of:

A: And your last name please?
B. Sicola.
A: F-I-C…? (spelling the letters)
B: *S::* ([es::]). *S* ([es]) as in 'Saturday.'
A: *Oh*, okay…

Gemination or segmentation of the of the sounds or syllables that cause the misunderstanding, as well as using spelling and orthographically oriented meta-language are equally common strategies to help the listener more accurately identify and rectify the problem.

Thus, it would also be informative to have a NS-NS baseline against which to compare negotiation strategies when participating on the map task. The lack of a NS control group for such comparison under experimental conditions is typical in L2 pronunciation research (Piske, MacKay, & Flege, 2001), and arguably in broader SLA research as well. A NS baseline could demonstrate whether or not NNSs provide each other with the same conditions through negotiations as NSs do. A stimulated recall session as done by Mackey, et al. (2000) could also shed light on participants' intentions and interpretations of critical exchanges, whether NS or NNS, adding further support in this direction. The greater the similarity between NS-NS and NNS-NNS negotiation patterns, the less concern researchers and practitioners should have regarding the value and authenticity of having two non-natives working together on language learning tasks, even when targeting pronunciation, and the greater the generalizability of the Interaction Hypothesis overall.

IMPLICATIONS

Although research has not been consistent in its definition of "acquisition," specifically whether pertaining to "highly accurate production on a more controlled task, or [...accurate production of] the structure in more spontaneous speech" (Hansen, 2004, p. 87), this study has demonstrated the potential for learners to push each other in a step towards acquisition in either condition. Under the conditions set forth in the study, it was found that learners can and do draw each other's attention to targeted phonological forms through an array of strategies, and modify their production towards more targetlike pronunciation. As many of their modifications were self initiated, it supports Shehadeh's (1999) claims that learner-based modifications are just as valuable if not more so than modifications in which the correction was provided by an interlocutor. Similarly, the more learners can be trained and encouraged to initiate and complete the repairs for themselves, the more they will approximate NS-NS interactional norms (Shehadeh, 1999). Thus, it is incumbent upon task designers (both researchers and practitioners alike) to establish task conditions that foster this type of dynamic, further reducing the belief in the need for NS interlocutors as an essential factor in interlanguage phonological development.

Another related implication is that the map tool can be equally – or even more – useful between *same-L1* interlocutors, if street names are adjusted to reflect only the phonemic contrast that causes problems for those learners. For example, if using such a task in an EFL context, such as in Japan, street names could be created so that all minimal pair names exclusively reflect the /s/-/θ/ contrast, without also including contrasts with /f/ and /t/. The findings may also hold potential applicability for work in the field of speech pathology, as a way to help students overcome a lisp by drawing attention to the contrast between /s/ and /θ/ and helping participants to distinguish these forms in communicative contexts through corrective feedback and pushed output.

Findings also lend further credence to the need for a shift in research and pedagogy alike in SLA. It strengthens the call for moving away from a predominantly product oriented view of "learning" to one that takes a stronger L2 processing orientation, particularly when conceptualizing L2 instruction (C. J. Doughty, 2003). This is as true for L2 pronunciation as any other branch of language development.

CONCLUSION

In conclusion, a goal of this study was to serve as a bridge between broader SLA interaction research and L2 phonological research, as identified in chapter 1. Findings of the study have provided evidence that SLA researchers need not shy away from doing phonologically targeted interaction studies, and that L2 phonology researchers might consider the value of exploring online modification of target phonemes rather than exclusively looking at phonological change from a post-hoc perspective.

With regard to developmental L2 phonology, acquisition of targetlike control of a form includes understanding of the existence of the form, neuromuscular ability to produce and perceive it on command (or withhold it when not required), and sociolinguistic competence in recognizing the communicative function of the form when applicable. Practitioners and researchers alike have the responsibility to help learners acquire these competencies in order to maximize their intelligibility and communicative competence. It is hoped that this study has taken a big step toward fulfilling this mission, and will inspire others to continue along the same path.

APPENDIX A: PRE-TASK

MINIMAL PAIR PRE-TASK ACTIVITY

Activity Instructions: (*Note: You may not look at your partner for this activity.)

1. From each numbered pair of sentences, you or your partner must choose either *sentence-a* or *sentence-b* and read it to the other person. The other person will listen carefully and try to understand which sentence was said.

2. If the listener thinks it was *sentence-a*, she/he will read *response-a*. If the listener thinks it was *sentence-b*, she/he will read *response-b*.

3. If the listener answers correctly, go on to the next number, but change roles each time. If someone makes a mistake, try to help each other fix the misunderstanding.

	Sentences	***Responses***
1.	a) Have you seen Beth today? b) Have you seen Bess today?	a) No, she's in New York this week. b) No, she's been busy lately.
2.	a) That tree is very thick. b) That tree is very sick.	a) That's because it's over 100 years old! b) That's because the insects have eaten the leaves.
3.	a) What an incredible oaf! b) What an incredible oath!	a) I agree, he is very clumsy! b) I agree, that's a hard promise to keep!
4.	a) She needs a bat. b) She needs a bath.	a) She can use mine for softball practice. b) I'll be out of the bathroom in a minute.
5.	a) That child is very mousey. b) That child is very mouthy.	a) I wonder why he's so shy. b) I wonder why he's so rude.
6.	a) They need to be re-tanked. b) They need to be re-thanked.	a) The old tanks broke. b) Then they will feel appreciated.
7.	a) This is the tense race. b) This is the tenth race.	a) Yes, I can't believe how much pressure there is! b) Yes, I can't believe we've won the first nine!
8.	a) We have thought about that a lot. b) We have fought about that a lot.	a) But we haven't come up with a decision yet. b) But we haven't come up with a compromise yet.
9.	a) It was a long and drawn-out debt. b) It was a long and drawn-out death.	a) I thought I'd never finish paying it off. b) I thought that movie scene would never end!
10.	a) I only have a pair of threes. b) I only have a pair of trees.	a) I am not good at playing poker. b) I am not good at gardening.

APPENDIX B: MAP TASK

INSTRUCTIONS AND MAP

“<u>Where in New Philadelphia is…?” Map Task Instructions</u>:

(*Note: You may not look at your partner’s map, and you may not make eye-contact with your partner for this activity.)

1. On the next page, you have a map of “New Philadelphia.” <u>You will be Partner A</u>, and your partner will be Partner B. Above the map, there is a list of popular tourist locations in New Philadelphia. You will need to give your partner directions to get to the places on your list, and your partner will give you directions to get to the locations on the Partner B List. One corner of each intersection is numbered.

2. For each place on List A, choose a street corner for its location. Write the number of the street corner on the line next to the place name on your list. (Example: If you want the Constitution Center to be at the intersection of Truce Alley and Fateful Way, you can write the number ***76*** next to the words “Constitution Center” on your list.) Choose a different number for each place.

3. When you are ready to “go sight seeing,” ask your partner for directions to the places on List B. These are the rules for giving and receiving directions:
   - First, the *receiver* must tell the other person where she/he will *start* walking. (Example: “How do I get to City Hall *from the intersection of High Pass Road and Booth Road*?”)
   - You can <u>NOT</u> tell your partner *how many blocks* to go. (Example: You can <u>NOT</u> say “Go three blocks south on Booth Road, and then…”) ☹
   - You can <u>ONLY</u> give street names and compass directions such as *north, south, east, west, right* or *left*. (Example: “From High Pass Road, walk east until Theme Park Drive. Turn south on Theme Park Drive and go to Mossy Hill Street. Then…”) ☺
   - You can <u>NOT</u> mention numbers on street corners when you are giving or receiving directions.

4. Finally, the person giving directions will lead the receiver to the intersection of streets where the location is, and ask what number is on the corner. (Example: “And finally, go south on Truth Alley until you reach Ticket Lane. The Liberty Bell is on the north-west corner. What number is it?”)

5. The receiver should then tell what number is on that intersection. If it is *correct*, then you can go on to the next location on the other person’s list, and switch roles. If it is *not* correct, go back to the starting point and try again.

Where in New Philadelphia is...?

Partner A:	Corner #	Location	Partner B:	Corner #	Location
	___	Constitution Center		___	Liberty Bell
	___	Reading Terminal		___	Art Museum
	___	Franklin's House		___	City Hall
	___	Penn's College		___	Italian Market

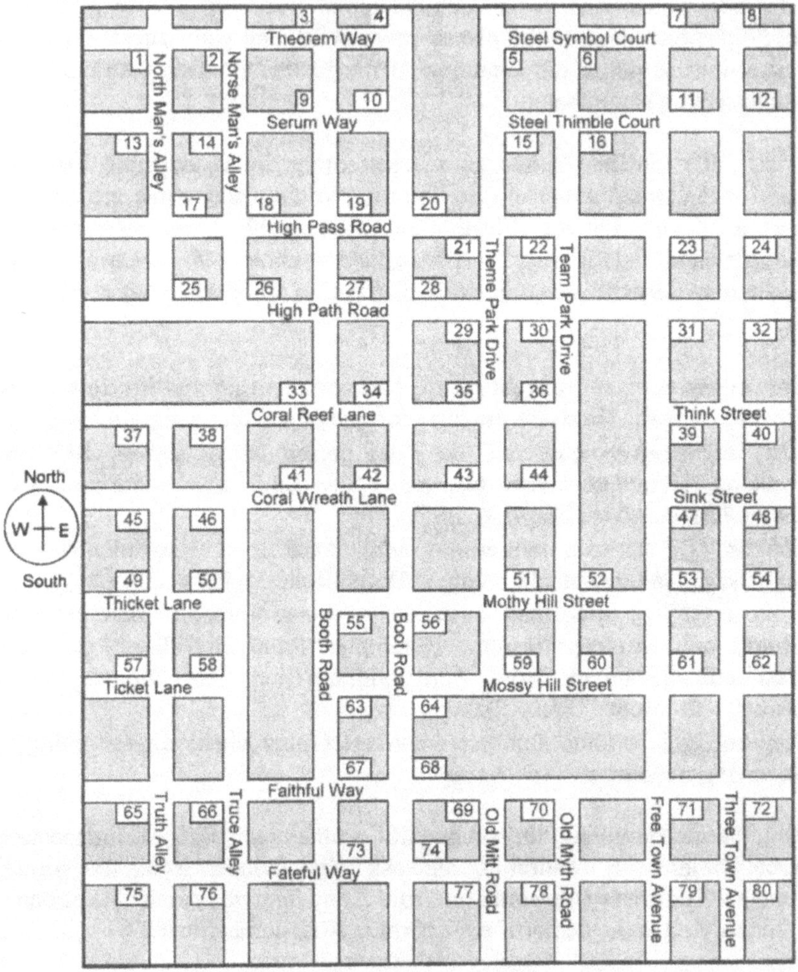

REFERENCES

Abrahamsson, N. (2003). Development and recoverability of L2 codas: A longitudinal study of Chinese-Swedish interphonology. *Studies in Second Language Acquisition, 25*, 313-349.

Archibald, J. (1998). *Second Language Phonology* (Vol. 17). Philadelphia: John Benjamins.

Avery, P., & Ehrlich, S. (1992). *Teaching American English Pronunciation.* Oxford: Oxford University Press.

Beisbier, B. (1995). *Sounds Great: Intermediate Pronunciation and Speaking for Learners of English*. Boston, MA: Heinle & Heinle.

Benrabah, M. (1997). Word-Stress-A Source of Unintelligibility in English. *IRAL, 35*(3), 157-165.

Bitchener, J. (2004). The Relationship between the Negotiation of Meaning and Language Learning: A Longitudinal Study. *Language Awareness, 13*(2), 81-95.

Bongaerts, T. (1999). Ultimate attainment in L2 pronunciation: The case of very advanced late L2 learners. In D. Birdsong (Ed.), *Second Language Acquisition and the Critical Period Hypothesis* (pp. 1330159). Mahwah, NJ: Lawrence Erlbaum Associates.

Bowen, C. (1998). Typical Speech Development: The gradual acquisition of the speech sound system. Retrieved November 5, 2006, from: http://www.speech-language-therapy.com/acquisition.html

Bruton, A., & Samuda, V. (1980). Learner and Teacher Roles in the Treatment of Oral Error in Group Work. *RELC Journal, 11*(2), 49-63.

Carroll, S. E. (2001). *Input and Evidence: The Raw Material of Second Language Acquisition* (Vol. 25). Philadelphia: John Benjamins.

Corder, S. P. (1993). A role for the mother tongue. In S. Gass & L. Selinker (Eds.), *Language Transfer in Language Learning* (pp. 18-31). Philadelphia: John Benjamins.

Crookes, G., & Schmidt, R. (1991). Motivation: Reopening the research agenda. *Language Learning, 41*(1), 469-512.

Dauer, R. M. (1993). *Accurate English: A complete Course in Pronunciation*. New York: Prentice Hall Regents.

de Bot, K. L. J. (1980). The Role of Feedback and Feedforward in the Teaching of Pronunciation-An Overview. *System, 8*(1), 35-45.

de Bot, K. L. J., & Malifert, K. (1982). The Teaching of Intonation: Fundamental Research and Classroom Applications. *TESOL Quarterly, 16*(1), 71-77.

Díaz-Campos, M. (2004). Context of Learning in the Acquisition of Spanish Second Language Phonology. *Studies in Second Language Acquisition, 26*(2), pp. 249-274.
Doughty, C., & Varela, E. (1998). Communicative focus on form. In C. Doughty & J. Williams (Eds.), *Focus on Form in Classroom Second Language Acquisition* (pp. 114-138). Cambridge: Cambridge University Press.
Doughty, C., & Williams, J. (1998a). Pedagogical choices in focus on form. In C. Doughty & J. Williams (Eds.), *Focus on Form in Classroom Second Language Acquisition* (pp. 197-261). Cambridge: Cambridge University Press.
Doughty, C., & Williams, J. (Eds.). (1998b). *Focus on Form in Classroom Second Language Acquisition*. Cambridge: Cambridge University Press.
Doughty, C. J. (2003). Instructed SLA: Constraints, compensation, and enhancement. In C. J. Doughty & M. H. Long (Eds.), *The Handbook of Second Language Acquisition* (pp. 256-310). Malden, MA: Blackwell Publishing.
Duff, P. A. (1993). Tasks and interlanguage performance: An SLA research perspective. In G. Crookes & S. M. Gass (Eds.), *Tasks and Language Learning: Integrating Theory and Practice* (pp. 57-95). Clevedon: Multilingual Matters.
Eckman, F. R. (2004). From phonemic differences to constraint rankings: Research on second language phonology. *Studies in Second Language Acquisition, 26*, 513-549.
Ellis, R. (1994). *The Study of Second Language Acquisition*. Oxford: Oxford University Press.
Ellis, R. (1999a). Retrospect and prospect. In R. Ellis (Ed.), *Learning a Second Language through Interaction* (pp. 233-257). Amsterdam: John Benjamins.
Ellis, R. (1999b). Theoretical perspectives on interaction and language learning. In R. Ellis (Ed.), *Learning a Second Language through Interaction* (pp. 3-31). Amsterdam: John Benjamins.
Ellis, R. (Ed.). (1999c). *Learning a Second Language through Interaction* (Vol. 17). Amsterdam: John Benjamins Publishing Company.
Ellis, R., Loewen, S., & Erlam, R. (2006). Implicit and explicit corrective feedback and the acquisition of L2 Grammar. *Studies in Second Language Acquisition, 28*, 339-368.
Finegan, E. (1999). *Language: Its structure and use*. New York: Harcourt Brace.
Foster, P., & Ohta, A. S. (2005). Negotiation for meaning and peer assistance in second language classrooms. *Applied Linguistics, 26*(3), 402-430.
Fromkin, V. (Ed.). (1980). *Errors in Linguistic Performance : Slips of the Tongue, Ear, Pen, and Hand* London: Academic Press.
García Mayo, M. d. P. (2005). Interactional strategies for interlanguage communication: Do they provide evidence for attention to form? In A.

Housen & M. Pierrard (Eds.), *Investigations in Instructed Second Language Acquisition* (pp. 383-405). New York: Mouton de Gruyter.

Gardner, R. C., & Lambert, W. E. (1972). *Attitudes and Motivation in Second-Language Learning*. Rowley, MA: Newbury House.

Gass, S. (2003). Input and Interaction. In C. J. Doughty & M. H. Long (Eds.), *The Handbook of Second Language Acquisition* (pp. 224-255). Oxford: Blackwell.

Gass, S., & Selinker, L. (Eds.). (1993). *Language Transfer in Language Learning* (Vol. 5). Philadelphia: John Benjamins Publishing Company.

Gass, S., & Varonis, E. M. (1985). Task variation and nonnative/nonnative negotiation of meaning. In S. Gass & C. G. Madden (Eds.), *Input in Second Language Acquisition* (pp. 149-161). Rowley, MA: Newbury House Publishers.

Gass, S., & Varonis, E. M. (1989). Incorporated repairs in nonnative discourse. In M. R. Eisenstein (Ed.), *The Dynamic Interlanguage: Empirical Studies in Second Language Variation* (pp. 71-86). New York: Plenum Press.

Gilbert, J. B. (1993). *Clear Speech: Pronunciation and Listening Comprehension in North American English (Student's Book)* (Second ed.). New York: Cambridge University Press.

Gorsuch, G. J. (2001). Testing Textbook Theories and Tests: The Case of Suprasegmentals in a Pronunciation Textbook. *System, 29*(1), 119-136.

Griggs, P. (2005). Assessment of the role of communication tasks in the development of second language oral production skills. In A. Housen & M. Pierrard (Eds.), *Investigations in Instructed Second Language Acquisition* (pp. 407-432). New York: Mouton de Gruyter.

Han, Z. (2004). *Fossilization in Adult Second Language Acquisition*. Clevedon: Multilingual Matters.

Hansen, J. G. (2004). Developmental sequences in the acquisition of English L2 syllable codas: A preliminary study. *Studies in Second Language Acquisition, 26*, 85-124.

Hulstijn, J. H., & Schmidt, R. (1994). *Guest Editors' Introduction.* Paper presented at the Consciousness in Second Language Learning. AILA Review.

Iwashita, N. (2003). Negative feedback and positive evidence in task-based interaction: Differential effects on L2 development. *Studies in Second Language Acquisition, 25*, 1-36.

Jenkins, J. (2000). *The Phonology of English as an International Language*. Oxford: Oxford University Press.

Koren, S. (1995). Foreign Language Pronunciation Testing: A New Approach. *System, 23*(3), 387-400.

Leeman, J. (2003). Recasts and second language development: Beyond negative evidence. *Studies in Second Language Acquisition, 25*, 37-63.

Long, M. H. (1996). The role of the linguistic environment in second language acquisition. In W. C. Ritchie & T. K. Bhatia (Eds.), *Handbook of Second Language Acquisition* (pp. 413-468). San Diego, CA: Academic Press, Inc.

Long, M. H. (2003). Stabilization and fossilization in interlanguage development. In C. Doughty & M. H. Long (Eds.), *The Handbook of Second Language Acquisition* (pp. 487-535). Malden, MA: Blackwell Publishing.

Long, M. H., & Porter, P. A. (1985). Group work, interlanguage talk, and second language acquisition. *TESOL Quarterly, 19*(2), 207-228.

Long, M. H., & Robinson, P. (1998). Focus on form: Theory, research and practice. In C. Doughty & J. Williams (Eds.), *Focus on Form in Classroom Second Language Acquisition* (pp. 15-41). Cambridge: Cambridge University Press.

Loschky, L., & Bley-Vroman, R. (1993). Grammar and task-based methodology. In G. Crookes & S. Gass (Eds.), *Tasks and Language Learning: Integrating Theory and Practice* (pp. 123-167). Clevedon: Multilingual Matters.

Lyster, R. (2004). Differential effects of prompts and recasts in form-focused instruction. *Studies in Second Language Acquisition, 26*(3), 399-432.

Lyster, R., & Ranta, L. (1997). Corrective feedback and learner uptake: Negotiation of form in communicative classrooms. *Studies in Second Language Acquisition, 20*, 37-66.

Macdonald, D., Yule, G., & Powers, M. (1994). Attempts to improve English L2 pronunciation: The variable effects of different types of Instruction. *Language Learning, 44*(1), 75-100.

Mackey, A., Gass, S., & McDonough, K. (2000). How do learners perceive interactional feedback? *Studies in Second Language Acquisition, 22*, 471-497.

Major, R. C. (1987). A model for interlanguage phonology. In G. Ioup & S. H. Weinberger (Eds.), *Interlanguage Phonology: The Acquisition of a Second Language Sound System* (pp. 101-124). Cambridge: Newbury House Publishers.

Major, R. C. (2001). *Foreign Accent: The Ontogeny and Phylogeny of Second Language Phonology*. Mahwah, NJ: Erlbaum.

Marinis, T. (2003). Psycholinguistic Techniques in Second Language Acquisition Research. *Second Language Research, 19*(2), 144-161.

Markham, D. (1997). *Phonetic Imitation, Accent, and the Learner*. Lund: Lund University Press.

Miller, S. F. (2000). *Targeting Pronunciation: The Intonation, Sounds, and Rhythm of American English*. New York: Houghton Mifflin Co.

Morley, J. (1991). The pronunciation component in teaching English to speakers of other languages. *TESOL Quarterly, 25*(3), 481-520.
Morley, J. (Ed.). (1994). *Pronunciation Pedagogy and Theory: New Views, New Directions*. Alexandria, VA: Teaching English to Speakers of Other Languages, Inc.
Neufeld, G. G. (2001). Non-foreign-accented speech in adult second language learners: Does it exist and what does it signify? *IRAL, 133-134*, 185-206.
Oyama, S. (1976). A sensitive period in the acquisition of a nonnative phonological system. *Journal of Psycholinguistic Research, 5*, 261-285.
Park, J. K. (2000). *The Effects of Forms and Meaning-Focused Instruction on ESL Learners' Phonological Acquisition.* Unpublished PhD Dissertation, University of Pennsylvania, Philadelphia.
Pennington, M. C. (1998). The Teachability of Phonology in Adulthood: A Re-Examination. *IRAL, 36*(4), 323-341.
Pennington, M. C., & Richards, J. C. (1986). Pronunciation Revisited. *TESOL Quarterly, 20*(2), 207-225.
Philp, J. (2003). Constraints on "Noticing the gap": Nonnative speakers' noticing of recasts in NS-NNS interaction. *Studies in Second Language Acquisition, 25*, 99-126.
Pica, T. (1984). Pronunciation activities with an accent on communication. *English Teaching Forum, 22*(3), 2-6.
Pica, T. (1988). Morpheme Data Analysis in Second Language Acquisition Research: Renewing an Old Debate and Raising New Issues. *ITL, Review of Applied Linguistics, 79-80*, 77-112.
Pica, T. (1994). Research on negotiation: What does it reveal about second-language learning conditions, processes, and outcomes? *Language Learning, 44*(3), 493-527.
Pica, T., Holliday, L., Lewis, N., & Morgenthaler, L. (1989). Comprehensible Output as an Outcome of Linguistic Demands on the Learner. *Studies in Second Language Acquisition, 11*(1), 63-90.
Pica, T., Kanagy, R., & Falodun, J. (1993). Choosing and using communication tasks for second language instruction. In G. Crookes & S. Gass (Eds.), *Tasks and Language Learning: Integrating Theory and Practice* (pp. 9-34). Clevedon: Multilingual Matters.
Pica, T., Kang, H.-S., & Sauro, S. (2006). Information gap tasks: Their multiple roles and contributions to interaction research methodology. *Studies in Second Language Acquisition, 28*(2), 301-338.
Pica, T., Lincoln-Porter, F., Paninos, D., & Linnell, J. (1996). Language Learners' Interaction: How Does It Address the Input, Output, and Feedback Needs of L2 Learners? *TESOL Quarterly, 30*(1), 59-84.
Piske, T., MacKay, I. R. A., & Flege, J. E. (2001). Factors affecting degree of foreign accent in an L2: A review. *Journal of Phonetics, 29*, 191-215.

Reed, M., & Michaud, C. (2005). *Sound Concepts: An Integrated Pronunciation Course*. New York: McGraw Hill.

Rickford, J. R. (1996). Regional and social variation. In S. L. McKay & N. H. Hornberger (Eds.), *Sociolinguistics and Language Teaching* (pp. 195-217). Cambridge: Cambridge University Press.

Robinson, P. (2001a). Task complexity, cognitive resources, and syllabus design: A triadic framework for examining task influences on SLA. In P. Robinson (Ed.), *Cognition and Second Language Instruction* (pp. 287-318). Cambridge: Cambridge University Press.

Robinson, P. (2001b). Task Complexity, Task Difficulty, and Task Production: Exploring Interactions in a Componential Framework. *Applied Psycholinguistics, 21*(1), 27-57.

Schmidt, R. (2001). Attention. In P. Robinson (Ed.), *Cognition and Second Language Instruction* (pp. 3-32). Cambridge: Cambridge University Press.

Schmidt, R., & Frota, S. (1986). Developing basic conversational ability in a second language. In R. Day (Ed.), *Talking to Learn* (pp. 237-326). Rowley, MA: Newbury House.

Schumann, J. H. (1976). Social distance as a factor in second language acquisition. *Language Learning, 26*(1), 135-143.

Scovel, T. (1969). Foreign accents, language acquisition, and cerebral dominance. *Language Learning, 19*, 245-254.

Shehadeh, A. (1999). Non-Native Speakers' Production of Modified Comprehensible Output and Second Language Learning. *Language Learning, 49*(4), 627-675.

Snow, C. E., & Hoefnagel-Höhle. (1978). The critical period for language acquisition: Evidence from second language learning. *Child Development, 49*(4), 1114-1128.

Spada, N., Lightbown, P. M., & White, J. L. (2005). The importance of form/meaning mappings in explicit form-focused instruction. In A. Housen & M. Pierrard (Eds.), *Investigations in Instructed Second Language Acquisition* (pp. 199-234). New York: Mouton de Gruyter.

Stokes, J. D. (2001). Factors in the acquisition of Spanish pronunciation. *ITL Review of Applied Linguistics, 131-132*, 63-84.

Swain, M. (1985). Communicative competence: some roles of comprehensible input and comprehensible output in its development. In S. Gass & C. G. Madden (Eds.), *Input in Second Language Acquisition* (pp. 235-253). Rowley, MA: Newbury House Publishers.

Swain, M. (1995). Three functions of output in second language learning. In G. Cook & B. Seidlhofer (Eds.), *Principle and Practice in Applied Linguistics* (pp. 125-144). Oxford: Oxford University Press.

Swain, M. (1998). Focus on form through conscious reflection. In C. Doughty & J. Williams (Eds.), *Focus on Form in Classroom Second Language Acquisition* (pp. 64-81). Cambridge: Cambridge University Press.

Swain, M., & Lapkin, S. (1995). Problems in output and the cognitive processes they generate: A step towards second language learning. *Applied Linguistics, 16*(3), 371-391.

Tarone, E. E. (1983). On the variability of interlanguage systems. *Applied Linguistics, 4*(2), 142-163.

Tarone, E. E. (1987). The phonology of interlanguage. In G. Ioup & S. H. Weinberger (Eds.), *Interlanguage Phonology: The Acquisition of a Second Language Sound System* (pp. 70-85). Cambridge: Newbury House Publishers.

Tomlin, R. S., & Villa, V. (1994). Attention in cognitive science and second language acquisition. *Studies in Second Language Acquisition, 16*, 183-203.

Varonis, E. M., & Gass, S. (1985). Non-native/non-native conversations: A model for negotiation of meaning. *Applied Linguistics, 6*, 71-90.

Weinberger, S. H. (1987). The influence of linguistic context on syllable simplification. In G. Ioup & S. H. Weinberger (Eds.), *Interlanguage Phonology: The Acquisition of a Second Language Sound System* (pp. 401-417). Cambridge: Newbury House.

Williams, J. (2005). Form-Focused Instruction. In E. Hinkel (Ed.), *Handbook of Research in Second Language Teaching and Learning* (pp. 671-691). Mahwah, NJ: Lawrence Erlbaum Associates.

Zuengler, J. (1989). Identity and interlanguage development and use. *Applied Linguistics, 10*(1), 80-96.

INDEX

DUISBURGER ARBEITEN ZUR SPRACH- UND KULTURWISSENSCHAFT
DUISBURG PAPERS ON RESEARCH IN LANGUAGE AND CULTURE

Herausgegeben von
Ulrich Ammon, René Dirven und Martin Pütz

Band 1 René Dirven / Yvan Putseys (Eds.): A User's Grammar of English: Word, Sentence, Text, Interaction - Part A. The Structure of Words and Phrases. 1989.

Band 2 René Dirven / Richard A. Geiger (Eds.): A User's Grammar of English: Word, Sentence, Text, Interaction - Part B. The Structure of Sentences. 1989.

Band 3 René Dirven / Wolfgang Zydatiß / Willis J. Edmondson (Eds.): A User's Grammar of English: Word, Sentence, Text, Interaction - Parts C & D. The Structure of Texts / The Structure of Interaction. 1989.

Band 4 René Dirven: (Ed.): A User's Grammar of English: Word, Sentence, Text, Interaction - Compact Edition. 1989.

Band 5 Martin Pütz / René Dirven (Eds.): Wheels within Wheels. Papers of the Duisburg Symposium on Pidgin and Creole Languages. 1989.

Band 6 Ulrich Schmitz / Rüdiger Schütz / Andreas Kunz (Eds.): Linguistic Approaches to Artificial Intelligence. 1990.

Band 7 Friedrich Lenz: Organisationsprinzipien in mündlicher Fachkommunikation. 1989.

Band 8 Luc Van Doorslaer (Hrsg.): Niederländische Literatur im Spiegel niederländischer Kultur. Aufsätze zur Gastprofessur von Prof. Dr. Marcel Janssens (Universität Löwen) in Duisburg, Sommersemester 1988. 1990.

Band 9 Frank Lüschow / Marita Pabst-Weinschenk (Hrsg.): Mündliche Kommunikation als kooperativer Prozeß. Sprechwissenschaftliche Arbeitsfelder. Festschrift für Elmar Bartsch. 1991.

Band 10 Susanne Niemeier: Ein Fall im Medienvergleich: Film- und Fernsehversion von "A Streetcar Named Desire". Beitrag zur Annäherung an eine Mediensemiotik. 1990.

Band 11 Paul Kent Andersen: A new look at the passive. 1991.

Band 12 Richard Kremer: The efficiency of English language teaching in smaller countries: Denmark. Basic English language teaching in Denmark and its wider context. 1991.

Band 13 Frank Lüschow: Sprache und Kommunikation in der technischen Arbeit. 1992.

Band 14 Günter Kellermann / Michael D. Morrissey (Eds.): Diachrony within Synchrony: Language History and Cognition. Papers from the International Symposium at the University of Duisburg 26-28 March 1990. 1992.

Band 15 Wim Waumans (Hrsg.): Mit fremden Augen. Niederländisch: eine Sprache, verschiedene Kulturgemeinschaften. 1993.

Band 16 Eberhard Klein: Konditionalität in didaktischen und pädagogischen Grammatiken des Englischen. Prinzipien zur Erstellung von Lehr- und Lerngrammatiken. 1993.

Band 17 Xiaoan Zhu: "Wenn sich das Gras bewegt, dann muß auch der Wind blasen!" Studien zur Metapher in der deutschen politischen Pressesprache – unter besonderer Berücksichtigung der China-Berichterstattung. 1993.

Band 18 Fritz Ponelis: The Development of Afrikaans. 1993.

Band 19 Martin Pütz: Sprachökologie und Sprachwechsel. Die deutsch-australische Sprechgemeinschaft in Canberra. 1994.

Band 20 Heiner Pürschel (Ed.); Co-Editors: Elmar Bartsch, Peter Franklin, Ulrich Schmitz, Sonja Vandermeeren: : Intercultural Communication. Proceedings of the 17th International L.A.U.D. Symposium. Duisburg, 23-27 March 1992. 1994.

Band 21 Dominiek Sandra: Morphology in the reader's mental lexicon. 1994.

Band 22 René Dirven: Metaphor and Nation. Metaphors Afrikaners live by. 1994.

Band 23 Ralph Bisschops: Die Metapher als Wertsetzung. Novalis, Ezechiel, Beckett. 1994.

Band 24 René Dirven / Johan Vanparys (Eds.): Current Approaches to the Lexicon. A Selection of Papers Presented at the 18th LAUD Symposium, Duisburg, March 1993. 1995.

Band 25 Michael Schloßmacher: Die Amtssprachen in den Organen der Europäischen Gemeinschaft. Status und Funktion. 1996. 2., durchges. Aufl. 1997.

Band 26 Johan Vanparys: Categories and Complements of Illocutionary Verbs in a Cognitive Perspective. 1996.

Band 27 Hideaki Takahashi: Die richtige Aussprache des Deutschen in Deutschland, Österreich und der Schweiz nach Maßgabe der kodifizierten Normen. 1996.

Band 28 Angela Heidemann: The visualization of foreign language vocabulary in CALL. 1996.

Band 29 Kazuma Matoba: Referenzperspektive in Sprechakten. Ihre Funktion und Entwicklung in der deutschen und japanischen Sprache. 1997.

Band 30 Olaf Jäkel: Metaphern in abstrakten Diskurs-Domänen. Eine kognitiv-linguistische Untersuchung anhand der Bereiche Geistestätigkeit, Wirtschaft und Wissenschaft. 1997.

Band 31 Birgit Smieja / Meike Tasch (Eds.): Human Contact through Language and Linguistics. 1997.

Band 32 Martin Pütz (Ed.): The Cultural Context in Foreign Language Teaching. 1997.

Band 33 Andrea Gerbig: Lexical and Grammatical Variation in a Corpus. A Computer-Assisted Study of Discourse on the Environment. 1997.

Band 34 Helga Bister-Broosen: Sprachkontakte und Sprachattitüden Jugendlicher im Elsaß und in Baden. Vergleichende soziolinguistische Untersuchungen in Colmar (Frankreich) und in Freiburg und Müllheim (Deutschland). 1998.

Band 35 Helga Bister-Broosen (Hrsg.): Niederländisch am Niederrhein. 1998.

Band 36 Alicja Sakaguchi: Interlinguistik. Gegenstand, Ziele, Aufgaben, Methoden. 1998.

Band 37 Benjamin Biebuyck / René Dirven / John Ries (Eds.): Faith and Fiction. Interdisciplinary Studies on the Interplay between Metaphor and Religion. A Selection of Papers from the 25th LAUD-Symposium of the Gerhard Mercator University of Duisburg on 'Metaphor and Religion'. 1998.

Band 38 Ulrich Ammon (Hrsg.): Sprachförderung. Schlüssel auswärtiger Kulturpolitik. 2000.

Band 39 El Hadj Ibrahima Diop: Das Selbstverständnis von Germanistikstudium und Deutschunterricht im frankophonen Afrika. Vom kolonialen Unterrichtsfach zu eigenständigen Deutschlandstudien und zum praxisbezogenen Lernen. 2000.

Band 40 Herman M. Batibo / Birgit Smieja (Eds.): Botswana: The Future of the Minority Languages. 2000.

Band 41 Harald Haarmann: Die Kleinsprachen der Welt – Existenzbedrohung und Überlebenschancen. Eine umfassende Dokumentation. 2001.

Band 42 Dirk Scholten: Sprachverbreitungspolitik des nationalsozialistischen Deutschlands. 2000.

Band 43 Riana Roos Paola: Pro-active Language Teacher Education in a Multicultural Society. 2001.

Band 44 Angelika Daniel: Lernerwortschatz und Wortschatzlernen im bilingualen Unterricht. 2001.

Band 45 Edel O'Halloran: Ist Mode englisch? Französische und englische Einflüsse auf die deutsche Mode- und Gemeinsprache im 20. Jahrhundert. 2001.

Band 46 Maya Khemlani David (Ed.): Methodological and Analytical Issues in Language Maintenance and Language Shift Studies. 2002.

Band 47 Martin Praxenthaler: Die Sprachverbreitungspolitik der DDR. Die deutsche Sprache als Mittel sozialistischer auswärtiger Kulturpolitik. 2002.

Band 48 Ulrich Ammon / Grant McConnell: English as an Academic Language in Europe. A Survey of its Use in Teaching. 2002.

Band 49 Birgit Smieja: Language Pluralism in Botswana - Hope or Hurdle? A sociolinguistic survey on language use and language attitudes in Botswana with special reference to the status and use of English. 2003.

Band 50 Carlos Inchaurralde / Celia Florén (Eds.): Interaction and Cognition in Linguistics. 2003.

Band 51 Andreas Ross: Europäische Einheit in babylonischer Vielfalt. Die Reform des Sprachenregimes der Europäischen Union im Spannungsfeld von Demokratie und Effizienz. 2003.

Band 52 Michael Anton Böhm: Deutsch in Afrika. Die Stellung der deutschen Sprache in Afrika vor dem Hintergrund der bildungs- und sprachpolitischen Gegebenheiten sowie der deutschen Auswärtigen Kulturpolitik. 2003.

Band 53 Martin Pütz / JoAnne Neff-van Aertselear / Teun A. van Dijk: Communicating Ideologies. Multidisciplinary Perspectives on Language, Discourse, and Social Practice. 2004.

Band 54 Yuko Sugita: Gesprächserwartungen. Eine kontrastive Studie über die Gesprächsführung in deutschen und japanischen Telefonaten. 2004.

Band 55 Eithne B. Carlin: A Grammar of Trio. A Cariban Language of Suriname. 2004.

Band 56 Maya Khemlani David (Ed.): Teaching of English in Second and Foreign Language Settings. Focus on Malaysia. 2004.

Band 57 Rita Brdar-Szabó / Elisabeth Knipf-Komlósi (Hrsg.): Lexikalische Semantik, Phraseologie und Lexikographie. Abgründe und Brücken. Festgabe für Regina Hessky. 2004.

Band 58 Claudia Kunschak: Language Variation in Foreign Language Teaching. On the Road to Communicative Competence. 2004.

Band 59 Allan Turner: Translating Tolkien. Philological Elements in *The Lord of the Rings*. 2005.

Band 60 Markus Motz (Hrsg.): Englisch oder Deutsch in Internationalen Studiengängen? 2005.

Band 61 Birte Kellermeier-Rehbein: Areale Wortbildungsvarianten des Standarddeutschen. Beiuntersuchung zum *Variantenwörterbuch des Deutschen*. 2005.

Band 62 Maya Khemlani David / Hafriza Burhanudeen / Ain Nadzimah Abdullah (Eds.): The Power of Language and the Media. 2006.

Band 63 Vít Dovalil: Sprachnormenwandel im geschriebenen Deutsch an der Schwelle zum 21. Jahrhundert. Die Entwicklung in ausgesuchten Bereichen der Grammatik. 2006.

Band 64 Sara Hägi: Nationale Varietäten im Unterricht Deutsch als Fremdsprache. 2006.

Band 65 Albert Weideman / Birgit Smieja (eds.): Empowerment through Language and Education. Cases and Case Studies from North America, Europe, Africa and Japan. 2006.

Band 66 Iraide Ibarretxe-Antuñano / Carlos Inchaurralde / Jesús-M. Sánchez-García (eds.): Language, Mind, and the Lexicon. 2007.

Band 67 Roswitha Reinbothe: Deutsch als internationale Wissenschaftssprache und der Boykott nach dem Ersten Weltkrieg. 2006.

Band 68 Fredericka van der Lubbe: Martin Aedler and the *High Dutch Minerva*. The First German Grammar for the English. 2007.

Band 69 Frank Polzenhagen: Cultural Conceptualisations in West African English. A Cognitive-Linguistic Approach. 2007.

Band 70 Augustin Simo Bobda (ed.): Explorations into Language Use in Africa. 2008.

Band 71 Johannes Eckerth / Sabine Siekmann (eds.): Task-Based Language Learning and Teaching. Theoretical, Methodological, and Pedagogical Perspectives. 2008.

Band 72 Laura Sicola: *No, they won't 'just sound like each other'*. NNS-NNS Negotiated Interaction and Attention to Phonological Form on Targeted L2 Pronunciation Tasks. 2009.

Band 73 Gerhard Stickel (ed.): National and European Language Policies. Contributions to the Annual Conference 2007 of EFNIL in Riga. 2009.

Band 74 Daniel Klaaß: Untersuchungen zu ausgewählten Aspekten des Konsonantismus bei österreichischen Nachrichtensprechern. 2009.

FSC
www.fsc.org
MIX
Papier | Fördert
gute Waldnutzung
FSC® C083411

Kolibri 360 GmbH
Ferdinand-Jühlke-Straße 7
99095 Erfurt, Deutschland
produktsicherheit@kolibri360.de

Druck:
CPI Druckdienstleistungen GmbH
im Auftrag der
Kolibri 360 GmbH
Ferdinand-Jühlke-Str. 7
99095 Erfurt